Rolling With The Waves
Our Parkinson's Journey

Rolling With The Waves
Our Parkinson's Journey

Claire Blatchford

Lorian Press LLC
Holland, MI 49424
www.lorianpress.com

Rolling With The Waves
Our Parkinson's Journey

CoverArt by Claire Blatchford
Book Design by Jeremy Berg

ISBN: 978-1-939790-23-1

Blatchford, Claire
Rolling With The Waves: Our Parkinson's Journey/Claire Blatchford

Library of Congress Control Number: 2019934541

First Print Edition February, 2019

Lorian Press LLC is a private, for profit business which publishes works approved by the Lorian Association. Current titles can be found at www.lorianpress.com.

The Lorian Association is a not-for-profit educational organization. Its work is to help people bring the joy, healing, and blessing of their personal spirituality into their everyday lives. This spirituality unfolds out of their unique lives and relationships to Spirit, by whatever name or in whatever form that Spirit is recognized. For more information, go to www.lorian.org.

*This book is dedicated to the Light
within each and all of us.*

One day he got into a boat with his disciples, and he said to them, "Let us go across to the other side of the lake."

So they set out, and as they sailed, he fell asleep. And a storm of wind came down on the lake, and they were filling with water, and were in danger.

And they went and woke him saying, "Master, Master, we are perishing!"

And he awoke and rebuked the wind and raging waves; and they ceased, and there was a calm.

He said unto them, "Where is your faith?"

And they were afraid, and they marveled, saying to one another, "Who then is this, that he commands even the wind and water, and they obey him?"

The Gospel of St. Luke 8:22-25 (RSV)

Table of Contents

Foreword

When I was six years old, I had a severe case of measles which caused damage to my auditory nerves. I did not totally lose my hearing as a result, unlike the author of the book you are holding, who became totally deaf at the same age due to the mumps. I did, however, become partially deaf.

Over the years, this condition has worsened. Like the frog who doesn't realize it is being cooked as the water around it is slowly brought to a boil, I didn't recognize what was going on. I could always hear sounds, but gradually, it became harder for me to decipher what people were saying. I found myself feeling isolated and not always comprehending the conversations around me.

Then I read one of Claire Blatchford's books, *Full Face*. It is a series of fictional letters written to a man who is slowly losing his hearing. In it, Claire describes the full spectrum of experiences and emotions that go along with becoming deaf (or in my case, deafer). This book was a revelation to me. I felt she was writing directly to me, for so much of what she described was what I was experiencing. Reading this book, I felt both seen and heard, and the result was liberating and healing. Through the stories she tells and the advice she offers in these letters, born of her own experiences of being deaf, she gave me emotional and mental tools for dealing with the challenges I was facing.

I feel this book, *Rolling with the Waves*, will do the same thing for those dealing with Parkinson's Disease, either as a patient or as a caregiver. With authenticity and honesty, Claire writes from the heart of her experiences in facing the challenges of living with PD as it has been manifesting in the body of her husband, Ed. In so doing, she gives us a book that is not only informative and helpful for anyone else navigating these same challenges but one that is healing as well.

As Claire herself points out in this book, there is a difference between *healing* and *curing*. One way to think of this is that curing seeks to restore what was, and it is wonderful when this happens. But healing is more mysterious and more profound. It takes us forward to what can be as a new pattern of wholeness. A wise friend once said to me at a time when I was dealing with cancer, "There is no healing power, but there are healing relationships." This simple statement helped me refocus from seeing myself as a "cancer patient" to seeing myself as a person in relationship with the world who also happened to have cancer in part of my body. I felt expanded, defined not by a specific disease but by my identity as a sovereign, spacious person. I felt reconnected to my world, to others, and to the healthy parts of my life, of which there were many—far more, actually, that the parts that were ailing.

This was deeply healing for me. I realized that "being whole" didn't mean simply being "altogether" or "fully functional" and without disease. It meant being open and engaged, a participant in life, a source of blessing as well as a recipient of such. It meant being present to life, the challenges and the joys.

This is the story that Claire eloquently tells in this book. She is honest about the ups and downs that she and Ed experience—their "rolling with the waves"—but underneath the surface where the waves rise and fall, you can sense the calm of the deep ocean itself, whether we call this depth "love" or "God," "faith" or "spirit". Though the book is about living with PD, it is even more about the resiliency and ability within each of us to tap these depths and thus to know the whole ocean—the wholeness of ourselves—and not just the part that goes up and down.

I don't see this as a "how to" book, though it is certainly filled with everyday wisdom about ways of coping with the challenges of Parkinson's Disease. Claire and Ed don't claim any special status as "teachers of how to deal with PD," and are certainly not setting themselves up as experts. I think of it more as a "who we are" book. Through the stories she tells, taking us into the ordinary events of their lives, Claire eloquently shines a light on the power in each of us to find new dimensions of who we are, no matter what we may be facing. Although this book is specifically about living with PD, the insights and wisdoms that Ed and Claire come to in their journey can be helpful in recognizing our wholeness in the midst of dealing with any unsought-for and unwanted challenge that life can present us.

Like *Full Face* did for me with my hearing loss, I believe this book offers the invaluable gift to anyone dealing with Parkinson's, either directly as a patient or indirectly as a caregiver, of being seen, heard, and understood. It leaves you feeling that you're not alone. This in itself makes this book worthwhile for anyone dealing with this disease.

But Claire does more than this. Through the largeness of her own spirit, she enables any of us to feel, whether PD is part of our life or not, that we are not alone, period. Claire is a beautiful writer whose skill with words and images I admire and envy, but she is more than this. In showing us the spirit we all have within us, connecting us to the wholeness of life, Claire is a healer, which makes this book a healer's gift.

January, 2019
David Spangler

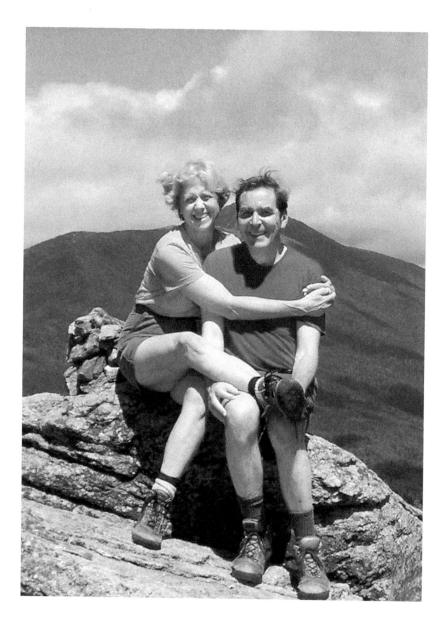

Ed and Claire hiking

Introduction

Living with Parkinson's disease is about learning to roll with the waves. This could be said about dealing with any chronic condition, any crisis when what we think of as "normal" is threatened or upset. I hear it from friends who after years of holiday letters packed full of happy yearly events have found themselves on the cancer path. I hear it often in the stories in my caregiver's support group. The first hint that one is no longer on solid, familiar ground may come when one senses that a loved one is looking, sounding, or behaving differently. Or the hint may be suggested by someone else: a family member, a neighbor, a coworker. Or it may come in a dream, or it may be far more than a hint, it may, when receiving a diagnosis, hit one quick and hard below the belt, like a totally unexpected tsunami.

Although it may be clear already, please keep in mind that I'm speaking here as a companion on this journey not as the one with the condition, although I'm speaking with the permission of the one with the condition. If you, as a person with PD or even as one close to someone with PD, are bothered by my manner of talking, excuse me. (I have chosen to refer to the condition as PD rather than Parkinson's throughout the book.) Ed and I have been married for over 50 years and—for better or for worse—the boundaries between us have become somewhat blurred. Sometimes, before it's even light, I wake up knowing Ed is unsettled, in the same way a sailor may sense, from the air or the feel of his boat, that he's heading into a stormy day. Though there's much solid ground beneath us the unknowns that come with PD are a constant presence in our lives. They are what have led me to the water metaphors you'll find throughout this account. Ed knows what I have written but, after much thought, chose not to be a cowriter. Writing—both the shaping of thoughts into words and the physical act—can for him be a laborious and frustrating process. He did, however, consent to composing the final chapter. Please feel free to read that chapter first if you want to hear his voice direct. I sometimes skip forward myself when reading a novel or the account of a journey and have a strong wish to take a peak at the outcome. But keep in mind that our journey certainly isn't anywhere near being over and we have no idea where it may take us next.

Even after a PD diagnosis has been made and absorbed, some sense of normalcy can return. The sun is still rising and setting, the stars are still there, the dog's still wagging his tail and coffee is still delicious. As a man we know, who also has PD, said shortly after his doctor identified the condition, "I realized I wasn't going to die today."

You continue onward, newly grateful for all you and your loved one have, happy to discover you can still do many of the things you've always done. Really, what does it matter if your beloved can't dot every "i" the way he or she used to? The sense of reprieve may stretch out or may be short lived. Suddenly, without warning, the sky can darken and the waves rise ominously as new symptoms emerge.

There's the feeling of being tossed out of every day life. You're less and less a participant. You feel yourself being forced into the role of observer. What do these symptoms mean? Who can you turn to for the best advice? How can all the information be absorbed? Sinemet. Rasagiline. Donepezil. The medications have unpronounceable names that sound like characters in science fiction. Where are you supposed to go from here? Until now you've been living with a pretty clear sense of probable destinations: retirement, travel, projects, even studies you might undertake. And now, while others your age seem to be enjoying their "golden years" here you are in the middle of an ocean and your physical well-being has become your central focus. You can lose the feeling of having a future.

You get used to this. After all, yes, the sun, moon, stars and more are still there and are, the more you look at them, amazingly beautiful, profoundly mysterious. You may have lost a certain form of mobility connected to definite, clear, outer goals, but you're catching sight of other forms of travel—travel that invites you into the Right Where You Are, as hinted at by William Blake in his poem "Auguries of Innocence":

To see a World in a Grain of Sand
And a Heaven in a Wild Flower
Hold Infinity in the palm of your hand
And Eternity in an hour…

And life goes on. You toughen up as new symptoms become the new normal. You can even speak with a bit of bravado, sometimes even with an air of authority. You may feel you're getting your sea legs, but are you, really?

Because, before you know it, another wave hits...

When you first got the diagnosis you may have had no interest at all in meeting others who are dealing with the same condition. Fact is, it can be scary to see the stoop, the lack of stamina, the shaking that can overtake those with PD: coming out of the doctor's office quietly, with long faces, sometimes one assisting the other. There are canes, walkers, maybe a wheelchair. You want your life to stay as it is, or was, for as long as possible. Then perhaps you catch a glimpse of yourself and your loved one in a store window as you're crossing the street together hand in hand. At first you don't recognize the two walking towards you. Wait a minute! Is that *your* own long face? Is that *your* grey hair? Isn't there a bit of a stoop in the one beside you? Yes, there's the tremor! Holy moly, it's us!

When you awaken to this mirroring, you might look away. Or you might begin to look more carefully at those others on their oceans who are finding their own ways of navigating. That's what happened to us. It wasn't a conscious decision, it just happened. It had to happen. You begin to look for the inner person who is there no matter what. You know you can't write a person off simply because he or she is declining physically, is inching his or her way out of life, or for any other reason that makes this other person different from you. This humbling revelation applies, of course, to your loved one and yourself as well.

The journey becomes more than just learning to roll with the waves: it becomes a journey of awakening to the soul within you and everyone.

Please note: most of the names have been changed to protect the privacy of our friends and helpers. We trust they will hear our admiration, affection and respect for them in the stories related in this book. We are very grateful they are a part of our journey.

Diagnosis

It's sometimes said that a diagnosis of Parkinson's is not so much a death sentence as a life sentence. The issue for people [with PD] is what we make of that life sentence. The remarkable Parkies I have met on my journey have convinced me of the importance of maintaining a positive attitude, even in the face of scientific setbacks. For as Tom Isaccs [a cofounder of the Cure Parkinson's Trust] once told me, "If you don't have hope in Parkinson's disease, you don't have anything."

Jon Palfreman, *Brain Storms, The Race to Unlock The Mysteries of Parkinson's Disease*

It was April 7, 2008, Ed's 64th birthday. We'd toasted our 40th anniversary the day before on April 6, but the real celebration of that event—with our daughters, their husbands, my father and his companion, our brothers and their wives—was coming that weekend. We'd figured out accommodations for everyone, lined up a babysitter for our young granddaughter, reserved space at a restaurant for dinner one night, and we had a list of suggested daytime activities to keep folks happy.

I was driving up the hill to our house with another round of groceries for the weekend and there was Ed, in his car, at one of the forks on our road. It was evident from his blinker he was heading home, too. But so early in the day? That puzzled me. Ed, an elementary and high school educator, had hardly ever, in our 40 years together, come home early from work. He was as closely wed to the hours of each school day and the school calendar as he was to me.

The other thing that caught my attention was the look on his face as I passed him with a wave. What was his face saying? What expression was that? I couldn't place it.

I'd known that morning that Ed was going to an appointment with a neurological specialist, not our primary care physician. His handwriting was becoming smaller and smaller and he'd developed a slight tremor in his right hand over several months. My boss at that time had what's called an essential tremor, which is a different thing entirely from the PD tremor. It had always been a part of Dave, it never got worse, and Dave didn't seem the worse for it, so I hardly noticed it any more. I guess this "not noticing it" or thinking about it at work made me not think much about Ed's tremor at home. In other words, I wasn't yet at the stage of checking out tremors online or in our medical encyclopedia.

On reflection, though, I *was* concerned about Ed's energy level. I felt fatigue in him not only often at the end of his work day but when we walked and hiked. We're avid hikers and were at that time out to climb the 47 New Hampshire peaks of 4,000 feet and over. I believed this fatigue was from his giving his all—every day, seven days a week—to starting up a charter school near our home in western Massachusetts. Yes, he worked with a small team of founders all great people but he was right then really carrying it all, emotionally as well as mentally. Others took vacations and long weekends but not Ed. This both worried and irked me at times. Part of that was necessity but Ed has always been super-conscientious. I will say I felt there was *something*—possibly cancer. But I didn't allow myself to dwell on it for long as I figured the school start-up tempo would shift into another, slower, gear at some point.

Shortly after Ed's car pulled up beside mine in our yard, he gave me the strange look again before forming the words, "The doctor said I have Parkinson's disease." That sent us straight to the internet and the medical encyclopedia.

Later, over the years, Ed has returned now and then to that moment and what he calls God's ironic sense of humor. As he sees it, "Isn't it strange that of the 365 days in the year I should get this diagnosis on my birthday, the one day when you think the world is behind you? I couldn't help but feel challenged. This was big! Was it a present? Hearing it on my birthday made me wonder if someone was saying, 'This is *not* what you think it is. It is *not* a disaster'."

Ed admitted later to feeling somewhat numb after the doctor told him he had PD. Others we know have used that same word when describing their reaction to the diagnosis.

Joan: *"I felt mostly numb, with some relief at having a clear explanation for the puzzling symptoms, especially the loss of smell.*

Liz: *"I was numb for days after I learned I had PD. I couldn't get up till late in the day."*

Later, too, we learned what is now common knowledge: how PD takes hold of an individual "decades before any tremors appear and continues wreaking damage throughout the brain until the end of life. This means that in addition to movement problems, people with Parkinson's... have to cope with a wide set of adverse symptoms from constipation to dementia." (*Brain Storms*)

So, the day we got the diagnosis was the day *we* became aware of PD. It was the day it entered our consciousness, though it was already in our lives. Indeed, it had been a part of our lives for some time. This is true of other chronic diseases as well—ALS, MS, cancer—and more.

After the naming, PD immediately began to become a presence in our day-to-day thinking. I think it's inevitable one finds oneself asking, "What, exactly, is causing this?" I believe we're wired to think in terms of "What—or who—is to blame for this?" It's like suddenly waking up and realizing one is on a path one hadn't realized one was on. A path that isn't likely to be a little jaunt around the park, and you think (or rather you feel), "Wait a minute, I had no idea I was here! I didn't ask to be here! When—where—did this path I'm on begin?"

So we began learning about possible environmental causes (was the water in our home, or any of the other homes we'd lived in, contaminated in some way?) other possible chemical issues (what about the lead paint in our first house?) and genetic causes (what about Ed's Uncle Hammond who we knew had had PD?). In connection with the last possibility, Ed had some genetic testing done about a year later with the hope of being able to alert our daughters to the possibility they, or one of their children, might find themselves on the PD path some day. The result of that testing was, thankfully, negative.

About two years after the genetic testing, when I mentioned it to a friend, he asked "Would you have done anything differently 42 years ago if you'd known Ed would be diagnosed with PD at age 64?" What I heard in his question was another question: "Would you still have married Ed if you'd known what was coming?"

My immediate response was, "No, I wouldn't have done anything differently!"

I was, in fact, offended by the question. As though one could pick another "healthier" husband (or wife, or partner) if one knew in advance what one was getting! I told my friend I believed in the love that brought

Ed and me together, "whether in health or in sickness, till death do us part." This is still the case.

But it was an important question for me to consider. A question that illuminated, rather than darkened, my life. It illuminated my life in the way that, when I'm working with pastels, the dark colors help illuminate the light colors. As a friend in my pastel class pointed out, the dark colors ground us, then the light colors can rise, and as they rise, lift, inspire, brighten and truly gladden us. If we're not grounded in the dark colors, the light colors make the pastel too wishful, insubstantial, unsteady, wispy.

Okay, you may say, but how does this apply to PD, which can be viewed as a pretty dark condition to begin with?

I am *not* saying I'm glad for the PD just because it makes me more appreciative of all Ed and I have—though it certainly does make me more appreciative. I'm saying that, even as I never know exactly what will happen when I'm doing a pastel painting, only by welcoming this not-knowing and whatever it may bring can a creative process unfold. As I move back and forth again and again between light and dark, dark and light, new possibilities emerge—possibilities I wasn't aware of when I began. So, whether one knows one is predisposed to PD or not, acknowledging that the darkness is *always* there in one form or another, is helpful. This acknowledgment helps to open the door to the light.

Here is a favorite quote from Alexander Graham Bell which I have returned to often throughout my life as a profoundly deaf person:

When one door closes, another opens;
but we look so long and so regretfully
upon the closed door that we do not see
the one which has opened for us.

Thoughts like this help keep the door open. They help me to find and then tap my own grit, grit I hadn't realized—and may still not always realize—*is* there. In every one of us.

Speaking of quotes that one can hold to, especially after diagnosis, or "re-diagnosis," for every time we go to the doctor we're hearing all over again, "Yes, you have PD", here's a quote I came across recently having to do with diagnosis. It's from *When Breath Becomes Air*, by Paul Kalanithi, the first hand account of a young doctor dying of lung cancer. It offers yet another way of thinking about, and dealing with, diagnosis.

*Patients, when hearing the news, mostly remain mute. (One of the early meanings of **patient**, after all, is "one who endures hardship without complaint.") Whether out of dignity or shock, silence usually reigns, and so holding a patient's hand becomes the mode of communication. A few immediately harden (usually the spouse, rather than the patient): "We're gonna fight and beat this thing, Doc." The armament varies, from prayer to wealth to herbs to stem cells. To me, that hardness always seems brittle, unrealistic optimism the only alternative to crushing despair.*

"We're gonna fight and beat this thing" *was* my response when we got the PD diagnosis. It was also my response when Ed got a prostate cancer diagnosis four years later. Are the hardness, brittleness and "unrealistic optimism" an instinctive emotional reflex? All I knew was that the life force within me would *not* be pushed down. It wanted—indeed, *needed*—to push back. Especially on behalf of the man I love.

With both diagnoses I felt as though a wall was unexpectedly growing up around us, cutting off the view we'd taken for granted all of our married lives: the view of a road meandering on and on, receding into the distance and with it the thrill and comfort of being able to discuss the unfolding of a journey, the freedom of being able to imagine what we wanted, and needed, to look for and work for. How fortunate, how privileged, we had been even if there were moments of upset and confusion as to where we were going. And now that feeling of the open road was being abruptly and rudely challenged.

It became a matter of not being overwhelmed by dark encroaching boundaries, of trying continually to define our life as a couple *on our own terms*. (This is true for each of us individually too.) We sensed that, if we did this, the other doors would appear and would open. And they have.

To speak plainly: for us there is not only the outer physical and medical path, but the inner spiritual path as well. They are finely interwoven. For example, when weary and discouraged we have found hope again and again in the Gospels, in the thoughts of David Spangler, a cofounder of the Lorian Association whose work is published by the Lorian Press, of Rudolf Steiner, an Austrian spiritual scientist, educator and founder of the

Waldorf School movement, and others whose writings I've listed at the end of this book. During these moments it is clear to me the open path is really an inner attitude rather than simply an outer reality. When I can sense this openness and the possibilities it brings within, and keep my eyes on it in faith and trust, I am able to recognize it without.

"Is there more PD today than there was, say, 50 years ago?" I asked a PD specialist seven years after the diagnosis. "There seems to be more of it because people are living longer" was her answer.

Her words reminded me of another point I'd picked up along the way: PD symptoms appear in *all* people as they age, it is potentially parked somewhere in everyone. Whether these symptoms congregate and link up in such a way as to lead to a diagnosis of PD is another matter.

My aim in writing about PD is not to offer a history of PD and the known medical and scientific responses to it; I believe the doctors, nurses, researchers and physical therapists committed to finding better treatments and possible cures are doing amazing work. My aim is to use our experience—Ed's, mine and that of some of our compatriots—to enter into the other half of the picture folks diagnosed with PD and their caregivers find themselves in. By "the other half" I mean the emotional, psychological and spiritual aspects, mentioned a minute ago, of living with PD. For healing—and the process of healing in PD has to be ongoing—is about *so* much more than just diagnosis, physical symptoms and the medical path one embarks on.

To return to April 7, 2008, I don't remember what I felt, except maybe relief that Ed wasn't saying the C word—yet! As mentioned earlier, Ed did have cancer and successful surgery for that four years later, and that's not a part of this story. Though the news was distressing there was also relief that a name had been given to our concern. What was present but invisible began to make itself visible in many ways, on many levels. In a sense we were out of the dark but the light was harsh and didn't flatter the landscape. This new landscape presented whole new sets of questions. The only thing that could soften or change the light was the hope I just spoke of. When low on hope, the view was stark and not very promising. But when we saw *with* hope we knew gratitude, deep, endless gratitude, for everything we had. This is still true.

After diagnosis we shifted our focus to prognosis—which, for us, meant the anticipated course of the disease, rather than recovery from it. When visiting the doctor, I couldn't help but think what a tough job it must be to be a PD specialist. Ongoing decline, rather than recovery, is *always* in the room. A doctor's task, as I see it, is not just to figure out what medications will help, how often, and so on, but to pass on pertinent information having to do with research, clinical trials, even, if possible, the efforts of different PD organizations (and there are many, all over the world). The good PD doctor helps the patient and his or her loved ones to feel part of the PD community. As a friend once observed, "One is inclined to feel alone. The art is to remain a team."

But, first, to return to our fortieth anniversary party. It was one of the most difficult events I've ever been through. I guess I was numb too. We'd only told our daughters about the diagnosis, because it didn't seem right to tell the others, some of whom had traveled a distance to be with us. Why put a damper on the celebration? Why not put this new trouble aside and plunge into the moment?

I've never been a good actress, can't pretend to be happy and full of fun when I'm not, so it was hard for me. I simply couldn't tell the PD to go away for a couple of days, it had stuck its foot firmly in the door and slipped inside. I remember being annoyed by my father's criticisms of the restaurant we'd picked. Heck, who cared if there weren't enough appetizers or we hadn't picked the best wine? Heck, too, to a relative who didn't come because of being too busy with "other things." Overnight the PD diagnosis had made a lot of former concerns sound like fluff! It still does that every now and then.

Why "fluff"? The challenge of the diagnosis, and the PD itself, is not only to one's perspective on life and what's important or unimportant; it is also a challenge to one's identity. And not once or twice but again and again.

I believe there is a part of us, or a being in us, that "knows" more than we may wakefully or consciously realize we know. How it knows, I don't know, but I somehow "knew" this diagnosis was coming, and it wasn't just because of Ed's tiny handwriting, the slight tremor or the strange walk. It was an an echo from an experience I'd had 38 years earlier.

It was in the fall of 1979, and we were living on Long Island. I was making a carrot cake for a birthday party we were having that evening, and a long-time friend, John, who was coming to the party, stopped by to leave something off. The children were playing in the living room while John chatted with me in the kitchen. I had awakened about 3:00 am that morning hearing the word *Parkinson's* in the middle of a dream, and for some reason remembered that right then. I hadn't mentioned the experience to Ed. I couldn't recall the dream, but could still hear the clear sound of that one word. What made it puzzling was that, hearing a spoken word, rather than lip-reading a spoken word, almost never happened when I was awake.

"Do you know anything about Parkinson's?" I asked John.

He shook his head. No he didn't know anything about Parkinson's.

"Are you afraid of getting it?" he asked.

"No, I just heard the word."

"Parkinson's?"

"Yes. Not 'Parkinson's disease,' just 'Parkinson's'."

John liked to think about the possible meaning of dreams. "So what do you think it means?" he asked.

I shrugged.

Then I told him that the first time I'd ever heard of PD was when I was a teenager. The mother of my best friend made weekly visits to a neighbor with PD, and took me along one time. My memory of this lovely, fragile, elderly gray-haired lady in a wheelchair is of her eyes. They were full—to the brim-- with words! Unspoken words, because she'd had an operation that had frozen the part of her brain connected to her hand tremors and silenced them, but the operation had taken away her ability to speak. Her eyes moved me deeply. I wanted to help translate what I was seeing into spoken words for her, wanted to be able to offer a response to whatever she was saying, but the nurse that day had other things in mind, so my visit was short.

As a deaf child I'd known what it was like to want to speak and not be able to—at least not as clearly as people expected. I'd had hours of speech therapy, and through that learned how eloquent the eyes can be, how they can say things in a second that the mind might need days, even weeks, to shape into words. Those few moments with the woman with PD called forth deep sympathy in me for those, individually and within the larger context of society, who may be viewed as the unheard or the voiceless.

Shortly after my visit, this woman died, but whenever I passed her

12

driveway I remembered her. And I realized as I remembered her again that morning while making that birthday cake how my first impression of PD had been formed then, my impression of PD as a confining, silencing, trapped condition.

I recall now also the ease with which I let the word *Parkinson's* go by after hearing it in my dream and having that brief conversation with John. I felt then, "If this is to be a part of my destiny, I'll deal with it when I come to it."

I was also feeling then the fullness of life at that moment, of being beyond the touch of physical decline, full of energy and youthful confidence (we were in our early thirties.) It did not occur to me that Ed might be affected by PD—then or later. My first thought was myself, and how, if I got it, that would be okay. Then I thought of my brother, as I'd noticed he sometimes had a very slight tremor of his head.

Was the word in my dream a premonition?

The *Merriam Webster's Collegiate Dictionary* (tenth edition) definition of *premonition* is: *1) Previous notice or warning. Forewarning. 2) Anticipation of an event without conscious reason. Presentiment. (A feeling that something will or is about to happen.)*

I googled *premonition* and was directed to Larry Dossey whose work in medicine and prayer I had read about once years earlier in his book *Healing Words*. I read on his website that premonitions are extremely common, in fact we're "hardwired for them." Dossey speaks of them as a part of our "original equipment," saying our bodies can respond to a future event before we're consciously aware of the coming or the actual presence of this event. It's the way our dog disappears into the basement a couple of hours in advance of a thunderstorm. He has his own internal weather channel and he wants to be underground, under something, when the lightning and thunder come.

Dossey adds that many premonitions arise out of close bonds, between parents, children, spouses, siblings, close friends and lovers. How often have you thought of someone and soon after received a phone call or email from that very person? You can invite premonitions in but not have them on demand, according to Dossey. And the best way to set the stage for them is to develop a discipline of quieting the mind, playing close attention to subtle messages from without and within and recording dreams wherein you sense you're getting premonitions.

While reading his take on premonitions I remembered others I've had over the years—and just about all of them turned out to be correct. But getting a premonition of something that would come to pass 38 years later?

Dossey says premonitions can reveal the presence of the spirit within us, can reveal "the presence of a timeless aspect of our consciousness," can "point like an arrow to an immortal, eternal aspect of who we are."

I found Dossey's words helpful and affirming, because for me there has always been what I'll call "the knower" and "the speaker of truth, comfort and love as well" within. Exactly who this knower and speaker is, I don't know. That's a question that has been with me for a long time. At the same time I know I don't *have* to know. I feel able to open myself to the mystery of it all rather than attempting to force this "timeless aspect of our consciousness" into a time frame or a neat, pat, intellectual explanation. That it *is* there, that it can provide truth, comfort and love when needed, strengthens my hope, the hope referred to in the quotation at the start of this chapter.

I believe I *was* having a premonition of some kind 38 years ago when I was awakened by the word, Parkinson's. Why? I don't know, but will go into this question in the chapters to come and see where it takes me.

Also, on reflection, I'm glad, really glad, that premonition was no more than that one word. I agree with the wonderful writer and poet Brian Doyle (who died recently. on the young side, of brain cancer), who wrote:

To see everything that would happen to you way
Into the future: that would be unmistakable hell.

From the poem "Astigmata"

14

The Thought Form of Parkinson's Disease

Early on, after Ed got the diagnosis, a friend warned us not to get caught up in the thought form of PD. I thought I knew what he meant but it's taken me ten years of living with PD to begin to fully understand. What's meant by "the thought form of PD?" Basically it is the definition of PD one may ascribe to.

It took me so long because I had to get ahold of the contemporary thought form of PD before I could begin to understand that the current definition of PD is by no means the final definition. And no matter how often the current definition changes or is updated, it will *never* be the final definition.

Here, for example is a definition of PD from the Parkinson's Disease Foundation:

Parkinson's disease (PD) is a chronic and progressive movement disorder, meaning that symptoms continue and worsen over time. Nearly one million people in the US are living with Parkinson's disease. The cause is unknown, and although there is presently no cure, there are treatment options such as medication and surgery to manage its symptoms. Parkinson's involves the malfunction and death of vital nerve cells in the brain, called neurons. Parkinson's primarily affects neurons in an area of the brain called the substantia nigra. Some of these dying neurons produce dopamine, a chemical that sends messages to the part of the brain that controls movement and coordination. As PD progresses, the amount of dopamine produced in the brain decreases, leaving a person unable to control movement normally.

The specific group of symptoms that an individual experiences varies from person to person. Primary motor signs of Parkinson's disease include the following.

tremor *of the hands, arms, legs, jaw and face*
bradykinesia *or slowness of movement*
rigidity *or stiffness of the limbs and trunk*
postural instability *or impaired balance and coordination*
Scientists are also exploring the idea that loss of cells in other areas of the brain and body contribute to Parkinson's. For example, researchers have discovered that

the hallmark sign of Parkinson's disease — clumps of a protein alpha-synuclein, which are also called Lewy Bodies — are found not only in the mid-brain but also in the brain stem and the olfactory bulb.

These areas of the brain correlate to nonmotor functions such as sense of smell and sleep regulation. The presence of Lewy Bodies in these areas could explain the nonmotor symptoms experienced by some people with PD before any motor sign of the disease appears. The intestines also have dopamine cells that degenerate in Parkinson's, and this may be important in the gastrointestinal symptoms that are part of the disease.

There's nothing wrong with this definition. Ed and I are familiar with many of these symptoms and their effects, although Ed also has symptoms that aren't mentioned in the above. To assume, though, that a definition like the one given is the *all* of PD was what my friend was warning me against. One's thought form, meaning one's idea, personal understanding or expectation of what a disease means, or is like, can rigidify in one's mind. It can become what one expects—and so, perhaps, what one gets. But, as we've found, the thought form of PD can and should stay malleable. It can change with time and experience. When you know little to nothing about a condition, you're open to allowing an outside story, fear, impression or definition to shape your understanding and response to it.

Perhaps one way to illustrate this is through my own experience with deafness. After I lost my hearing overnight from the mumps at age six, my parents had certain very definite ideas about deafness. As it was obvious from day one that I couldn't understand them when they spoke, my deafness meant the possibility of their not being able to communicate with me. So they were intent on finding ways for me to hear again and to continue communicating verbally with them.

My father researched hearing aids, but none of were powerful enough at that time to help me. He also asked around about medical research. I believe something like what he hoped for back then appeared later in the form of the cochlear implant. (I got one when I was 67.)

Years after I'd gone to college and become a teacher of the deaf, my parents told me that they'd visited a school for the deaf early on and were so horrified by the speech of the children, that they decided I would "become deaf" if I went there. So I remained in public school and I didn't know another deaf person (except for my grandmother) until I was in my twenties. They wondered why, after I'd been mainstreamed all my life, I wanted to become a teacher of the deaf. I tried to show them the beauty of American Sign Language—how a simple, single gesture or two could convey many sentences of meaning, but it was always, in their eyes a primitive language, if a language at all. Proof of the rightness of their view was how few used it, and how spoken language was the norm. So they adhered all their lives to their thought form in regards to deafness and ASL.

Their approach to my schooling was bold, for deaf children were, at that time, nearly always put in institutions for the deaf. My father was certain scientific research would find a way to bypass defective ears but it didn't happen fast enough for him. In his thought form of deafness, medicine and technology combined would find a way to fix my damaged nerves so my brain would be able to get sounds again. It didn't occur to him, though, that just getting sound isn't the all of hearing. Memory, comprehension, synthesis, as in the combining of several modes of physical and subtle perceptions, are all important parts of the act of hearing. Simply providing amplification of sound doesn't mean one automatically hears normally and is able to comprehend what one is hearing.

Another aspect of my parents' thought form of deafness lay in the fact that they never let go of their view of me as the hearing daughter they had known between birth and six years of age. They were constantly reminding me that I was perfectly fine. After I got my first hearing aid at age 12, they told me when I had difficulty understanding or making myself understood that I wasn't really paying attention or trying hard enough. Their thought form of deafness held me to a standard that was both helpful and hurtful; helpful in that I always thought of myself as "normal" because they'd known me as "normal," and hurtful in that they weren't interested in learning what it was like to be deaf. Their thought form of what it means to hear was based on their own experience as hearing people.

Diagnosis can—without one being fully aware of it—plunk one down in a certain thought form of PD. I have seen people with PD who look totally flattened by the disease. And I know Ed *is* flattened at times by PD, yet I also know we can't afford to let a single apparently scientifically correct definition of PD monopolize our experience of PD. The truth of the matter is we are far more than just a physical brain that

17

enables us to operate this way or that way. Scientists today are excited about neuroplasticity—in this context the ability of parts of the brain that are still healthy and functioning to take over tasks damaged parts of the brain can no longer manage. Yes, our brains are more complex, vital and supple than was assumed even a decade ago. But I believe there's even more to it than that.

Rachel Naomi Remen, MD, in her book *Kitchen Table Wisdom: Stories That Heal* expresses simply and beautifully the importance of not letting our understanding of a disease be governed by a thought form:

> *A label is a mask life wears.*
>
> *We put labels on life all the time. "Right," "wrong," "success," "failure," "lucky," "unlucky," may be as limiting a way of seeing things as "diabetic," "epileptic," "manic-depressive," or even "invalid." Labeling sets up an expectation of life that is often so compelling we can no longer see things as they really are. This expectation often gives us a false sense of familiarity toward something that's really new and unprecedented. We are in relationship with our expectations and not with life itself.*
>
> *Which brings up the idea that we may become as wounded by the way in which we see an illness as by the illness itself. Belief traps or frees us. Labels may become self-fulfilling prophecies.*
>
> *In my experience, a diagnosis is an opinion and not a prediction. What would it be like if more people allowed for the presence of the unknown, and accepted the words of their medical experts in this same way?*
>
> *Like a diagnosis, a label is an attempt to assert control and manage uncertainty. It may allow us the security and comfort of a mental closure and encourage us not to think about things again. But life never comes to a closure, life is process, even mystery. Life is known only by those who have found a way to be comfortable with change and the unknown. Given the nature of life, there may be no security, but only adventure.*

Sudden Tears

I could barely make it till Ed went to work before the tears began. (This was a few weeks after the diagnosis.) Did he notice then how hurried my goodbye kiss was, and how I was on the way up stairs as he went out the door? I didn't think so and hoped not. I understand now that I needed to do this grieving on my own without him feeling he was the cause of it.

My study looks out over the garage. I'd stand by the window, the tears streaming down my face, as he backed the car out and then headed down the driveway. I couldn't control the flow of these tears. I didn't cry aloud, really; there was just this gentle sobbing and this steady stream wetting my face, my hands, my neck, and sometimes my clothes. It might continue for 10 to 20 minutes while I tried futilely to hold it back, mopping it up with tissues.

I felt helpless, scared and altogether embarrassed when this happened, which, in the beginning, was always suddenly. I didn't know what was going on. Was I having some sort of breakdown? I could barely see when I was weeping and I definitely did not want to be seen. It was as though something in me was dissolving. So I hid, in my study, in the woods near our house with the dog, behind sunglasses if I was in a public place, or in the car.

Then I began to know when the deluge was about to come. I felt a pressure, a kind of buildup building up behind my eyelids. If I was in public I was certain people could see it coming on. Surely my mouth was pulling down, giving me away. Surely my eyes looked as leaden as they felt. Surely I croaked like a frog when I spoke.

When the tears had passed I would feel washed out, if not washed away—and very wobbly. I'd bury my face in a wet washcloth, warm water (yes, more water) on red eyes. Through it all I felt the need to "hold on"—to a calm exterior, to the belief that everything would be okay, answers would be found, we'd take care of each other, and so on. Then, gradually, I'd move on into the day, less wobbly, feeling a bit the way one feels as one is emerging from an illness—a bit ethereal, not fully here, sensitive to loud sounds and the helter-skelter of everyday life.

This went on for what seemed like quite a while.

There's a saying in a little book, *Light on the Path*, written down by Mabel Collins, which often came to mind when I wept in those weeks after the diagnosis:
Before the eyes can see they must be incapable of tears.
I took those words to mean I had to get beyond being so sensitive. How could I be attentive to Ed if I dissolved so easily? And why, really, was I weeping? For him? For us? For myself? If I could see clearly, bravely, then I'd be able to see what to do. Ed and I had, after all, had 40 wonderful years together—and we had wonderful daughters, a bright little light of a granddaughter, dear friends, caring family, a devoted dog and a beautiful home. I needed to remember all that. Why should I expect things to continue exactly as they always had? And I really, truly wanted, after being helped by Ed in so many ways for 40 years as a deaf woman, to be of help to him. It was my turn.

This self-talk didn't help much. I was still subject to the tears.

I sought distractions, took on additional projects at work, walked hard, swam laps often. Meanwhile Ed sought out a second opinion with a well-known PD doctor in his eighties in New York City, recommended by a cousin.

On the way to see Dr. C negotiating a confusing interweaving of congested highways, we got a flat tire. It was pouring rain. Ed carefully steered the car off the road onto a small patch of concrete. I helped change the tire, praying all the while we wouldn't get hit.

We mentioned the flat to the doctor when we came in on the late side. After guiding Ed through a very thorough examination that confirmed the "textbook" diagnosis of the first doctor and talking us through the medical options he looked intently into Ed's face when they shook hands in farewell.

"You drove all the way down from western Massachusetts," he said warmly, "changed a flat tire on a busy highway in the rain, and… you got here!"

That comment carried us all the way home. It was such an important reminder of what we *could* still do, *were* still doing.

Curiously—for a while—remembering those words called forth *more* tears. Dr. C had probably seen many heartbreaking cases of PD during

20

his lifetime, had walked beside many patients from diagnosis to death, yet he knew the most potent medicine of all was hope.

We never saw him again. I don't even know if he's still alive. But his white hair, his brisk yet kindly manner and the way he shook Ed's hand are still very much alive in me. Memories of this sort are sources of strength.

The tears still came, once or twice a week. I didn't tell Ed about them. One day when the sudden tears were a bit too sudden, I sat down at the computer and wrote my friend Michael for help. It was the best thing I could have done. I still have his email response:

There IS sadness and helplessness — they are real feelings that exist in the world, in us, in the air. The only way out may be through. That is, have you ever had the chance to allow the tears, sobbing, sadness, helplessness to fully have their way with you, so they can go through their changes? They may be like the first movement of a symphony that will endlessly re-play if you don't let it play through the subsequent movements. This would mean truly allowing the feelings/tears full sway, but all the time being willing for the current of feeling to take on a new course or a new hue. You would encounter the fear of being swept away, but I don't think you would be.

What he said was *exactly* right for me: a steadying hand on my arm in the midst of the deluge, a much-needed remedy, a way to go. Above all, the reassurance that it was okay to weep, and weep, and weep. I need not be ashamed of what I was feeling. He was giving me permission to flow with these bottled -up feelings.

"Sadness", "helplessness" — having the feelings named by someone else made them more valid. It was a diagnosis of another sort, a necessary diagnosis. A disease never affects just one person in a family, or, for that matter, one person in a circle of friends, or a community, or a town, or... the world! Everyone is affected.

Even as I felt myself to be affected by the medical diagnosis, *my* body, not just Ed's, was being affected, as evidenced by the tears. As I moved through the sudden tears, I couldn't help but marvel at the unflinching honesty of the physical body. While my mind struggled to make sense of what Ed's diagnosis meant, where to get the best information, who to believe, how to respond to all the suggestions from well-meaning others, what might be in the cards for us further down the road and so on, my body was doing its best to deal with the rush of emotions being called up.

The weeping didn't automatically stop when the feelings were acknowledged. But that it rained every now and then didn't mean I was being swept away. My feet were still on the ground. Thus the tears became messengers rather than intruders, messengers I could see from the window approaching the house before they knocked. The tears became visitors and—eventually—friends.

But that was later.

While I was struggling with sudden tears, Ed was, of course, struggling, too. (Did he experience tears too? He says no.) We heard a fair amount of talk of depression as being a normal consequence of diagnosis, and being a normal symptom of PD as time went on. All the talk around and about PDs *does* get depressing, no question of that.

But someone pointed out how depression and sadness are two quite different things. And that rang a bell with both of us. Neither Ed nor I wanted to think of ourselves, or be thought of, as depressed, but sadness we could relate to. Before the diagnosis we'd talked about what we wanted to do when we retired: world travel, service work, maybe even the Peace Corps. I'd been getting invitations, before the diagnosis, to visit educators of the deaf in foreign countries to see what they did for their deaf children. That interested me greatly.

Then suddenly such talk and dreaming were pushed aside, or so it felt. The unknowns around PD seemed formidable. So-and-so, who'd been diagnosed a year and a half ago was now using a walker. We remembered Mr. G, another educator, who had PD. He'd come to dinner at our house a few years earlier and I recalled how rigid and expressionless he appeared. Michael J. Fox wasn't quite the inspiration we wanted, though, bless him, he certainly is going far and furious with the life and the response to PD that he's chosen for himself. And he'd had to face the first challenges at a much younger age than Ed. We knew we were lucky next to him. But really, what does "luck" mean when you're experiencing sudden tears? Who wants to be told what they're experiencing is nothing beside what someone else is going through, or has been going through for the longest time already? I needed to meet and take in my own grief; that's what the tears brought home to me.

And now, almost eleven years later? Yes, I still weep at times, especially when I haven't gotten the sleep I need. And the older I get, the more important is the quality, not just the quantity, of sleep. There are times I'm not sure whether the tears are friends who have overstayed their welcome, or friends who have been transformed into angels.

I know it's presumptuous to think of rewriting that line in *Light on the Path*, but here is what I'm learning:

Before the eyes can begin to see they must be washed by tears.

Now I don't think I would feel quite right if my eyes were incapable of tears.

Seeing

Yes, I saw the slight tremor ten years ago but it was when Ed and I were walking that I realized something was seriously off. I couldn't see anything specific; I just knew something was different. But what? Not until after the diagnosis did I realize what it was. For at our first meeting together with the neurologist, she pointed out how Ed's right arm wasn't swinging as he walked. His left arm swung, but not the right one. It hung by his side like a limp empty sleeve.

Of course! How could I *not* have noticed that? How could a person who had never met my husband (the doctor) see that right away whereas I, who had at that time been with him for 40 years, couldn't? When had it stopped swinging? All of a sudden or gradually?

We can see but not see. We can think we are seeing and not see at all. It's quite mysterious. That I hadn't noticed that Ed's right arm had dropped out of the walk reminded me of another occasion when something changed in Ed's outer appearance and I didn't register it right away.

I'd gone away for a couple of days to a conference, and when I returned Ed looked thinner, lighter, more compact. Puzzled, I asked, "Did you get a haircut or something?" Ed laughed and laughed. Then he ran one finger slowly over his upper lip. He'd shaved off his mustache when I was away! I simply hadn't noticed the absence of the mustache, and I think of myself as a pretty observant person! I was mortified. (His kiss *had* been different without that mustache!)

Seeing—and not being able to see—the man I married, love and wake up with every morning is brought home to me over and again through the lens of PD.

What do I mean by that? There are, of course, the changes: the right arm hanging by his side, the altered walk, the thinness, the stooped shoulders, the PD mask, the miniscule handwriting, the fact that it takes longer—and longer—for him to type emails, get dressed, go places, do just about anything.

In the early days I made note of some of the things I was seeing:

I watch
your right foot
become more hesitant.
As if little eyes
in your toes
are closing
one by one
11/10

Your face says less
or else
says it wrong.
You can look stern,
distant,
angry,
but there's no anger
in your eyes.
So this is what they mean
by "The Mask."
10/10

What bothered me
a year ago—
the hunch of shoulders,
the slow bowing over
beneath a heavy hand,
like the bending,
of our beloved birch
in the ice storm—

My eye now accepts it—
An unfortunate happening.
Yet I cannot
but seek still
the upright shine
of unalloyed dignity.

For it *is* there
no matter what.
Come storm and rage,
come ice,
come wind,
you can bend my back
but you won't uproot my love!
3/11

Then I stopped looking, stopped seeing. Who wants to spend one's time making note of or counting the changes? Sometimes the sheer number of changes is confusing rather than challenging. You realize, deep down, that you have to let go of seeing–not just the outer seeing but the inner holding to what you believe and want to see.

I realize now, this *has* to happen. Because PD isn't only about visible outer changes in the physical body, it's about emotional and spiritual changes as well. To begin to tune in to these inner changes—and, it is hoped, accompany the person with PD on his or her journey—one *has* to go beyond the outer changes.

For example, it's of no help to Ed if I'm upset when we're walking and his gait is affected by the PD. The issue is not my upset, sadness or impatience, which is not to say those emotions are invalid. The issue is being open to and finding what I call the light flow within every moment. As Ed is stumbling along I can acknowledge the upset I feel and the frustration Ed must be feeling. As I witness what's happening and give thanks for it, rather than being repulsed by what I'm seeing, it is possible to become aware of a different way of seeing. I sense myself connecting with this lighter, less weighted, less tense and draining, way of seeing. I do not "see" some mystical light, but inwardly I feel a lightening of the heavy feelings and, because of that, a change in the way I am able to perceive what's going on. I may see outwardly how Ed is walking more on his toes than his heels and how this makes him more hunched over, less upright, less balanced, more prone to stumble and fall. I may point this out to him and he will straighten up and his step will change. Or he may see the difficulty himself and seek a different way of meeting it, such as pulling in his jaw which, in turn, makes him more upright.

This is a very common example—a physical therapist would call him on it if she was with us. That we are able to change our emotional response to what is happening *as* it is happening is what is essential. When we do this we are more able to roll with the waves rather than being overwhelmed or pulled under by them.

The spiritual changes are subtle and inward. One meaning of the word "spiritual" is "incorporeal." That these changes may not be seen with the physical eyes doesn't mean they're any less real. One can sense one's resolve, resilience, flexibility, humility, hope and even one's sense of humor being strengthened as one goes along. *Those* are spiritual qualities. *Those* are at the core of what I mean when I speak of spiritual changes.

There was the question early on about "coming out." It is about being seen, asking to be seen in a certain way or announcing something that may not yet be obvious. Whom to tell? How? When? I admire how willing Ed is to let others know, while it's also evident he doesn't want attention drawn to himself.

"Did they notice anything?" "Did anyone say anything?" he'd ask—and sometimes still asks—after family get-togethers or gatherings with friends. And he will look relieved when I say no. Whew! He made it through another meeting without the PD symptoms being detected or being glaringly obvious. (I know that sense of relief. Getting by, slipping by in the "normal" world of everyday interaction is part of the job when you're deaf.)

Ed can also be appreciative when I say, "Yes, they asked about you." I can see he is glad, though he would never say it, that others see it isn't always easy and he is pushing back. Don't we congratulate folks when they complete a road race? Every day is a road race for Ed, and some days the race is uphill and quite a bit longer than other days.

I see too how he can be doubly appreciative when people who care ask him directly, "How are you?" The way it is said can mean so much. To Ed it says, "You really see me!" Sometimes the quality of the sympathy moves him, and I see tears in his eyes. We're also both aware of those who never ask any questions, ever. I wonder if they don't notice he's walking with a cane, or if they're afraid of asking. Afraid of interfering in something private. Afraid to learn something they don't want to have to think about. I know that one, and so does Ed. I know there are limits to my own sympathy. Another bombing on T.V.? Sorry, I can't watch another one tonight.

It became clear after the diagnosis how much some people wanted to share with us how *they* saw PD. There was one woman who said that, by acknowledging the presence of PD we were enabling it, were not looking with the eyes of God at the perfect human being, and only by looking in this way and holding close to Scripture could healing occur. Another woman spoke of Mind over Matter: I'm unable to describe how this works so won't say any more. I heard a fair amount of talk about diet being a possible cause of PD—likely because I'm the cook at home—and there were others who said they saw PD as a necessary part of Ed's karma. What they meant was that the PD is playing a major role in his life path, to make him wiser or as atonement for something he might have done in a previous life.

Ten years ago these views from well-meaning people called up quite a range of emotions, from amazement, to disbelief, to anger and annoyance. We still occasionally receive unsolicited opinions and advice of this sort. But I've found, in the long run, how such encounters can actually strengthen one's resolve to follow one's own inner compass. Thankfully Ed and I are either going by the same compass or we get very, very similar readings from our inner compasses! Meaning this suggestion isn't that helpful, while that one *is* something to ponder. We pretty much see eye-to-eye on this journey we're on.

I find it easy to see when being in the public eye makes Ed contract, how he's suddenly eager to get out of crowded, hard-to-move-through spaces without freezing up. He may need to sit down, to pause for a few minutes, as if getting through these spaces can be as strenuous as climbing a mountain. When I've asked him how he sees himself, not just in the mirror but in the faces of others as they look at him, his responses have ranged from dismay at the stoop of his shoulders and his lack of energy or facial expression, to resolve to get a better sense of what helps and doesn't help, to modestly exclaiming, "I'm doing pretty good—I'm hanging in there!" It's inevitable that every now and then he compares himself to others with PD and asks if I'm in agreement with his assessment. More often than not I feel he's on target, though a bit too hard on himself. And when he is hard on himself, he is more easily discouraged.

Seeing him—seeing the noble, courageous core that *is* Ed—is much like catching a glimpse of the blue sky on an overcast day. Yet this doesn't necessarily always have to do with how he's standing or how energetic his walk, although the place he's in inwardly is usually reflected pretty

29

clearly outwardly. There have been times when I wonder if he's faking a show of resolution and good cheer, and I suspect the answer to that lies more in the quickness or slowness of his response than in the words themselves. Sometimes he says, "You know me too well. With you I can't fake anything," and I'm both glad and not glad when he says that. Why *not* glad? Because there are times when I too, want to fake it, get away from it, could actually sit in front of the TV for a couple of hours of mindless looking-at-something-else.

An affirmative and quick "I'm okay!" is more convincing than a hesitant "I'm fine."

Ed said once that the sedentariness of PD is what bothers him the most. He doesn't want to be seen as sedentary, less active, less energetic, slowing, unemployed, aging.

Heck! Isn't that true for me, too? Don't I make these endless lists of things to get done and over-schedule things at times? It's as though outer activity, briskness, nimbleness, industry, busyness is the purpose of life, the only valid way to be seen.

Speaking of sedentariness, we went to a PD dinner and presentation once by a new doctor in the area who was eager to make his services known. We went not because we were doctor shopping but out of curiosity and because a free dinner was being offered at a well- known restaurant. We'd never been to this restaurant, so why not try it out this way and see if this doctor had new PD information to share?

When we got there I could see some folks eagerly examining the menu and the contents of the appetizer table, while others hovered over the information table covered with printed brochures. It was pretty evident who was there to shop—meaning who was newly diagnosed—and who was there to eat.

We wound up at a table with a woman I knew and her parents (her mother had PD) and a couple we'd never met before. That woman, whom I'll name Sue, was with her husband, whom I'll name Tom.

Sue was quite clearly in a state of frantic resolve. Her expressions, motions and words all said, "I'm going to take notes on everything, I'm going to get all the information I can, I'm going to get this bloody PD into a corner and into a cage. I *will* contain it!"

Tom's PD was clearly beyond containment.

He was bent, not just at the shoulders but all the way through. He walked with a walker and the walker looked as if it rose up out of some hole in the ground. He just barely moved.

Sue had to remind him to keep pushing the walker. It had a basket on the front with his meds and a bottle of water to take his meds, and I think I noticed a knitted hat for his head, and who knows what else. Sue had an oversized pocketbook with a notebook sticking out and pens clipped in an outer pocket and her cell phone and iPad and, again, who knows what else.

We were already seated when Sue quickly parked herself beside one of the free spots at our table and helped Tom shift over from walker to chair which he sank into while leaning heavily on the table.

When Tom sat down, I got the feeling we were looking at a helpless mass of a man—exactly what anybody with PD fears. I'm sure many in that room wondered what we too were wondering. Did Tom have dementia as well as PD? I felt we were also looking up close, almost *too* close, at a marriage in danger of unraveling sometime soon.

Tom, whose face was almost at table level, proceeded to eat his potatoes, green vegetables and chicken (which Sue had cut for him.) Then he stuffed rolls into his mouth. When the doctor hosting the event began his talk just a few feet away from our table, Tom began drifting off. At one point his head was on the table. Sue kept nudging him awake. Each time she elbowed him awake, he'd look at her, then briefly over at the doctor, then he'd look around for something more to eat.

I was shocked by what I was seeing. They could have been in the midst of a particularly bad day—yes, that happens to us too—and when it happens Ed and I both retreat from society to some degree. We *have* to retreat and regroup. The fact that neither Sue nor Tom acknowledged or interacted with any of us at the table, or apparently anyone else, is what upset me. It was as though the whole event—the dinner specially—was merely a stop at a gas station.

I may sound judgmental here. I know I was responding to what I was seeing with my ordinary every day eyes and God knows what there was to see beneath and behind this difficult situation. Maybe some day Ed and I will find ourselves unable to connect with others who may wish to offer help, but I sure hope not! I hope we can always reach out to others. I hope we can hold close to our sovereignty, our best, most gracious, and appreciative selves.

When Ed's cousin told us her husband didn't want to tell others about his PD diagnosis, we understood, because it can be a while before you're ready to be identified with that crowd. You want life to keep on as usual. We were also sad, because we now know what a huge relief it can be to be with others with PD, not to feel the need to hold one hand with the other in order to quiet, or hide a tremor. Theo said it was though the light had gone out of Ben, and she asked Ed to please communicate with him. Which he did. Ben thanked Ed and they have had a few more conversations since then. It is clear –as with any situation—that different strokes work for different folks.

Having PD makes it easy to detect others who have it, even when it's in the early stages.

Ed gives me a nod—or I give him one—in the direction of this or that person in a store, in the airport, on the street, someone who's walking ahead of us or has just passed us. Another one. We exchange a look and a nod, and silently send a blessing his way.

I said, "his way." Whether that's because we've heard that more men than women have PD, or because I'm accustomed to looking primarily at Ed, I don't see PD as often in women.

But we do know several women with PD: Joan, the two Elizabeth's, and Nancy in our PD dance class. I see the PD mask on each of them. I feel deep concern for Joan particularly as she lives alone and is getting thinner and thinner, the tremor in both hands making her look like a leaf that's going to get ripped right off a limb and blown away when the next big storm blows through. Yet I can hear—and sometimes see—the great reserves of strength she is drawing upon.

She is a doctor by profession, a pediatrician, and her husband died suddenly before she was diagnosed with PD. She's said more than once how glad she is that her beloved Paul was spared her diagnosis and her condition now. For me, there's something overly self-sacrificing in this but if her belief helps keep her going, who am I to comment on it? Perhaps he *is* with her now, is able to offer a purer form of help and comfort than he could have offered if he was still alive. I know *I* have received help from those on the other side many times. (I attempt to describe my experiences in my book, *Experiences With The Dying and The Dead*, published in 2007.)

I see how Joan goes immediately for her cell phone during the break in dance class. She's often on it just before class, too, and then again soon after the class ends. Confirming, strengthening and checking out her connections with whom? Her two sons? (They live at a distance. I gather they aren't overly protective of her and wonder if she is trying to spare them just as her husband Paul, has been spared from the picture of PD up close.) Her close friends? I see how she responds right away to my emails and how she's alert to what's going on in the news day by day. I see her love of poetry in the poems and quotes at the end of her emails. Her selections are beautiful, hopeful, full of concern for the future of her grandchildren—indeed, our whole world! She isn't in complete agreement with their upbringing (we have compared notes and laughed together at our personal annoyances and puzzlements in this department) yet is completely into the role of being a grandmother. I hope they realize how grand she is.

In Joan I see a steady day-by-day affirmation of the need to stay involved in the world and to find ways to give to it—because it is in giving that we receive. And it is in giving that we remain connected, and when we connect we find healing.

Another woman in the PD dance class—Liz, or Lizzy—is painful to look at. She sits like a Raggedy Ann doll, flopped over, clothes hanging on her, sometimes revealing her underwear, hair disheveled, swollen legs and swollen feet clad in tight black slippers. All of her hangs down. I see how clothes sometimes just hang on Ed and Joan—but, underneath, neither of them is merely hanging. The PD hasn't wrung them out to that extent. The eyes of this Liz burn and beg. In all honesty I keep my distance. I greet her when she comes in, I wave at her when she looks at us across the room, and say good bye when her husband wheels her out, but I can't bring myself to get involved. It's not only because I find it hard to hear and understand what she is saying. I have to protect our boundaries. That's all I know. Ed comes first. Again, that's all I know.

The PD mask has been one of the hardest things of all for me to accept. When I lost my hearing, shortly after turning six, I had to learn to read faces. Quickly! I learned to smile before the person I was looking at smiled to let that person know I was fully present, especially if I hadn't heard what he or she might have said. As my mother was always urging me, "For God's sakes, *respond*! Show people you're here! Or they're going to walk right by you - you'll never be a part of anything!"

33

I read faces, then lips, then faces, lips, movements, gestures, dress, color, pace and more, all woven together. I learned how the eyes can say one thing while the mouth is saying something quite different. I hated Halloween and the masks that came with it because the masks weren't readable. For me that was scary, for a mask usually has one expression only—grin, grimace, smile, frown, blank—even if the eyes behind/within it may be alive with questions or commentary, even if the person's tone and words may convey quite the opposite of the mask.

In the beginning, before I was fully aware of extent of the PD mask, I reacted emotionally to it. I was annoyed at Ed's lack of enthusiasm, shocked by Nancy's look of blank misery, horrified by the self-involved smirk of a guy we sat with at a PD dinner. Surely, with a *little* effort, a little self-reflection, a person could be alert to, could change, his or her expression. Like putting on a bit of makeup, making sure you don't have spinach on your teeth, neatening your hair, and so on. In the world of appearances we are generally aware of and responsible for the faces we're presenting to the world. We're generally participating in the unspoken exchanges that come with these appearances: replying to, or ignoring invitations, or advances, accepting or judging others before we've even communicated.

But I began to understand Ed didn't have the control he wanted over his facial expressions and was aware of that. I was reminded of being deeply upset, rather than amused, as a child by a scene in one of Marcel Marceau's shows. In this scene the famous mime was stuck with a smiley face—a look he couldn't get off no matter how hard he tried. And it looked, as he wrestled with it, as though there was the danger of his whole face falling apart. It was scary.

How others responded to the PD mask came home to me with time. Our eldest granddaughter asked her mother if her grandfather was annoyed by her. And so our daughter, and her daughter, talked to Ed with greater awareness of the PD mask.

About then, I remembered a conversation Ed had had, shortly before the PD diagnosis, with one of our future sons-in-law. In the middle of this exchange Thor exclaimed, "You're upset with me—I see it on your face!" Ed sounded as hurt as Thor by this unexpected comment. Later, looking back, I thought, "Ah! Of course! The PD mask was visible even then..."

Through the lens of PD, there are other things to see, too, like the kindness in the face of the very overweight clerk at the supermarket whenever Ed and I go through. This guy is young, maybe 20, way to young to have to bear so much weight. You can't even see where his chin ends and his neck begins. I find it painful to look at him. But I see the glad way his eyes greet Ed. It's my guess Ed chooses, when by himself, to go through this cashier's lane knowing he won't be impatient while Ed fumbles to get out his credit card or the coins from his pocket spill onto the floor. And he will lift the bags and put them in the cart for Ed even before Ed has paid, even if it's a task for him to get himself around the counter to the shopping cart. I have seen it happen. I have seen the two men exchange simple blessings in their, "Goodbye, good day." So much more than what I think I am seeing is often taking place.

Sure, there are the impatient cashiers and the folks with the "What's the matter with you?" frown. Who knows what others may read into Ed's tremor. Alcoholic? Drug addict? Crazy old man? But, I know there is kindness everywhere. "After you, Sir." "Can I help you?" "How are you doing today?" I know Ed has felt burdened by it at times, being singled-out, being seen as fragile, weak, needy, disabled, aging. Yet someone who needs help not only brings out the goodness in strangers, but *their* need as well. The need to reach out, meet another, and in such meeting also meet oneself.

In dance class I see Ed anew in the mirroring we do together. The familiar fingers that are his only—doing household repairs, working with wood, wielding a chisel, sculpting clay, lifting rocks, starting up the chain saw or the lawn mower—come alive in the air, offering the weaving movements his body longs to make. His hands become seals, diving down into depths, shooting up into heights, curving round, then down, then up again. I can barely keep up with those two seals, now separate, now together, now suddenly folded in prayer as, with a little nod, he hands the movement over to me, asking me to carry it on. I'm so glad for the freedom of his hands in these brief yet always surprising movements. In the PD dance class I see here and then there, in the shrinking bodies of the others, not only seals but birds, butterflies, bouncing balls, bending trees, sprouting leaves, blooming blossoms, pacing cats, peeing dogs, charging bulls and more. With music, the limits of PD are able pushed back and bottled-up dreams, fears and exclamations are released.

In dance class I see too, not only how hard the foot movements are for Ed to bring consciousness to, but how his feet are getting more like

35

roots, uprooted roots still trying to hold onto the earth, trying to help him keep his balance so he won't topple over. How pale his feet look, how downright tenacious and precarious at once.

Often when we are together at gatherings, at the dinner table, at parties, Ed gives me a look, a look I am only beginning to understand and accept. It is the look of a man having difficulty finding the thoughts, the feelings and the words he would share if this shadow was not being cast over his consciousness. He says he feels he has nothing to share and is embarrassed and ashamed by that, that the conversation is moving too fast for him to latch on to it and go with it. His eyes say, "I need to step back from this rush of words and thoughts, I need to go back into a quiet, private place. Please speak for me. Please be my connector."

My eye now seeks out the upright, the quick and strong, the full dignity of the human stance in others—how effortless it can seem! How noble, pure, perfect! We do not know what we have when we have it, particularly in our youth. And when we have it, how could it possibly be any other way? How could there ever be a time when it might be otherwise? When it might come to end or be halted abruptly? It is as though the perfect human form within us is not meant to have any end. Even if it ends without we go on seeing it within, like a phantom form.

Emily, the young lifeguard at the pool, has a face that troubled me for ages because seems to be so lacking in expression, in empathic self-forgetful response. Yet her body is fit, strong and upright. Her strokes are smooth and powerful and display a certain inner knowing in right and graceful movement. It's strange feeling this frank admiration for her body in its ease, beauty, dignity, when I don't like her personality much, when I wish she could be more aware of others. I have to chuckle as I swim, how ironic she's a lifeguard. Maybe, just to see what else there is to see in her, I should fake a drowning some time!

Now I understand those hungry looks I received when I was a young woman and went on Sundays to visit my grandfather in the nursing home. My mother thought the old men excelled at dirty looks. I didn't know what she meant. It was so easy to give a smile of recognition, a wave of goodbye. Why *not* give generously when the appreciation was so evident? Now I know that we can, and do, find strength when we see the wholeness and beauty of another. I can feel when I am grasping at what I see, grasping with longing, wistfulness, even outright envy. And

36

I can feel when I am accepting what I see with admiration, respect and gladness. The feelings are altogether different. The first way of seeing makes me shrink within. The second makes me expand.

Does Ed see this way too?

Now my eye is sharpened to the presence of beauty and inner wholeness of being.

Mike has it though he has no legs from the knees down and hobbles on his prostheses. His face is a sun offering warmth to all. His face calls forth sun smiles in return-- even a small uncertain smile from Emily, the lifeguard.

I see—and treasure—the moments when Ed responds to his own decline with humor; when, to shake off the festination (freezing of gait), he attempts to turn jerky movements into dance steps, into silliness, even into magic. A little twist of the hand into the air, a hop called up out of a stumble and...presto! There's a lightness in the act of defying gravity, in the ability to thumb a nose at lurking despair.

I see daily how, no matter how often I say, "We're in this together" — and we are—Ed's experience of PD is his and mine is mine. And the task of love is to weave them together, to weave them into something altogether new.

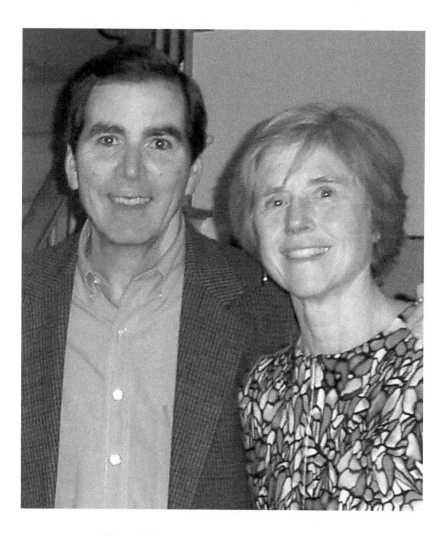

Ed and Claire shortly before the diagnosis

Stepping Out

Gone are the days when we'd step out the door early in the morning, packs on our backs, the dog sniffing round and round in excited circles, and spend the whole day on the trail, or on the road. That's my idea of a vacation: stepping out, stepping from one world into another, from inside to outside, even if we've known that outside—be it a mountain range or a woodland trail—for almost as many years as we've been married.

One day outside can be a vacation, the way one perfect apple, peach or pear can be a meal. There was always something new, something different to be found, seen, experienced when stepping out for a hike: an enormous rut in the road from the storm the night before, drops glistening on grass blades in a shaft of sunlight, a patch of foxgloves I'd never noticed till then, a blue-gray dragon of a cloud reclining on the peak we'd decided to climb.

As I learned from my White Mountain days with Ed, hiking and walking are very different experiences. Not that I'd never climbed a mountain before—I had, as a kid in the French Alps with my parents—but I hadn't, till I met Ed, had the chance to really meet mountains through feet, eyes and hands.

Hiking is different from walking in that I have to figure out— sometimes very quickly—what can hold my weight, if a tree root is strong, if a stone is slippery, if my boot will fit in a certain space, in short if I can trust the land and my body to carry me forward, upward, downward, sideways, yet ever onward. My relationship with the earth, and my body, too, becomes closer, more intimate, than when I'm just walking. It's amazing to me how, when hiking, eyes, hands and feet work together—not only reaching down into the land I'm coming into contact with but reaching—even "touching"—out ahead as eyes tell the body, "Don't go there—go here" or "Twelve inches over is too many. Six would be better." I feel myself to be more deeply *in* my body, especially when the terrain is unclear or treacherous.

Watching Ed move ahead of me on the trail, I marveled often at the confidence in his movements. He didn't worry the way I did when leaves were wet, and when he tripped, he would right himself easily, nimbly, as if dancing. While I panicked mid-stream when crossing a river, he'd stand on the opposite side grinning at my discomfort. Or he would re-cross the river to escort me, like a knight out of the Arthurian legends, to the far side. Yes, I marveled at this confidence he had and how he didn't think twice about it. After all, he'd been hiking for years and had worked in the AMC huts in the White Mountains, backpacking 100 pound loads of food up and empty gas cylinders back down.

And now? Now when we hike in the Audubon sanctuary near our home—which is much tamer than the White Mountains, the Canadian Rockies, the Grand Canyon and other places we've hiked—Ed often uses a cane or hiking poles. I'll confess I was, for the longest time, a snob when it came to any form of hiking or walking equipment to make things easier. Was amazed when, in the 1970's, we began meeting hikers on the trails in the White Mountains with trekking poles. Some of these folk reminded me of Daddy-Longlegs that had been brushed off a wall and had landed upside down on the floor. It was the way the poles some times seemed to flail about in the air as the hikers climbed, especially when they had a pack on their back. I was accustomed to using my hands to grab at rocks, shrubs and trees and to assist me downwards on my rear end. I don't remember Ed using his rear end often but mine has served me very well all these years.

Then Ed tore the meniscus in one knee, had to have surgery and I saw, as he recovered, how wooden walking sticks friends had given him were not just handsome but obviously useful objects. My view of walking equipment began to change. This change was hastened when, six or so years ago, the PD started to affect Ed's balance and an interesting assortment of canes, made of different materials, with curved, straight and padded handles, popped up in our lives. Some had belonged to my mother or father. One has a flashlight to help him walk at night. Another, a personal favorite, was carved by a cousin. It's pale ash with a spiraling body and, at the top, the arched neck and head of a horse. The arched neck is the handle. If you look closely when Ed is using it, the horse's round eyes peer out from between his fingers.

Now, even with a cane or a walking stick—Ed sometimes pretends his walking stick is his Wizard's Staff—I can see the Hiker's Confidence guiding him. I believe this confidence is a deep body understanding, a knowing, we are born with. Some fit right into it, almost unconsciously, the way you might say a person is a "born" athlete, while it may take others time and effort to connect with it.

When Ed hikes with this confidence, it's as though his body is greeting the path and each stone he steps on or tree he steps over. His body is fully present. This ease makes it look as though the landscape is reciprocating, is saying, "Welcome, neighbor!" This is something I've noticed with young children playing outdoors with total absorption, and also with farmers and gardeners deeply attuned to the earth they're tending. There's this wordless dialogue going on between their physical bodies and the soil, the trees and plants, water, sun, air, the elementals and more. Movements, touch, gestures, glances, all speak.

I'm not sure I'd be noticing these things as frequently and with such wonder if not for the PD. When PD slips into the picture, Ed's stride is broken. His gait can become stumbling, sometimes followed by the festination usually where there are sudden turns or the path is momentarily obscured. I see how his focus has to shift away from being fully present to the land to his body and getting it from here to there. Home again, he sometimes sinks onto the sofa or his rocker, exhausted

I so admire Ed for wanting to hike despite all this, for wanting to take the smaller, less trod paths that branch off the established trails, for wanting—maybe *needing* is the better word—to check out the lady's slippers in the spring, the beaver dam, the Wolf's Den which is a scramble, even for me.

To hike according to *Merriam Webster's Collegiate Dictionary* means "to rise up; to move, pull or raise with a sudden motion, to work upward out of place." This definition implies effort, *exertion*. A hike for some may have nothing to do with the outdoors, may mean simply getting up some stairs. I nod at this definition, because PD really *is* a hike. An ongoing effort, a continual exertion to be upright, not bent, not hunched over. It's no mere ramble, stroll, or saunter.

I salute my daily companion, traveler, intrepid hiker!

Walking is really quite different from hiking. Most of the time I walk without thinking about what I'm doing, without giving my surroundings the kind of attention I freely offer, or am forced to offer, when hiking.

As a child I got in the habit of going out walking (back then parents, fortunately, allowed kids to do this) accompanied by the family dog. Subconsciously I was *walking away from* a lot of things that upset me: speech therapy, demanding, worried parents, homework, confusion, and more. Sometimes when Ed says he's going out walking, I wonder if he doing that, too. Is he trying to walk away from, or walk off, the festination that often plagues him inside, indoors? And, yes, the festination sometimes seems to get left behind. When he returns there's the feel of deepened breath to him and sometimes an air of discovery. Maybe he's worked out something that's bugging him, maybe he's got a hideout I don't know of, like my den deep within a forsythia bush when I was seven years old.

Early on, we kept hearing from several different directions about the importance of exercise. "Use it or lose it" was the refrain from Ed's first PD doctor. What she meant, though she didn't put it this bluntly, was, "Keep moving or the PD will swallow you up and one day you'll find you can't move." Wanting to move is not a problem for Ed. He's never been a couch potato. We heard about the benefits of biking, from Claude, who's had PD for about 20 years and bikes about 2,000 miles a year. We also heard a fair amount about tandem bikes. A well person sits in the front seat and sets the pace, a hard and fast pace, forcing the person with PD, on the back to bike hard and fast. It was discovered that such exercise, strenuous by comparison with how a person with PD might ride alone, could make the PD symptoms recede—at least for a while. Ed was interested, but I wasn't. I have difficulty hearing cars coming from behind when on a bike, and we live on a hilltop. I have zero interest in huffing and puffing my way up our hill on any bike, let alone a tandem bike!

Then Ed heard about a clinical trial for people with PD at the Center for Neuro Rehabilitation at Sargent College of Boston University. They were studying the benefits of using Fitbit technology to set individual goals for regular walking. It was a natural fit. We drove the two-plus hours to meet the physical therapists overseeing the trial: attractive young women with great sympathy, energy and humor. First came some tests to set a baseline, then came some exercises to loosen up stiffening PD limbs, then instruction on how to operate the Fitbit and the small laptop they loaned Ed. His mileage, as registered by the Fitbit was recorded daily on his laptop and their computers too. He sometimes walked eight to ten miles a day, and they were checking in with him at a distance—cheering him on, giving him feedback when he needed it. Ed received some delightful encouragement from the program during those two years. For instance:

"Congratulations, you have now walked around the coast of Florida!"

(To which he replied, "Without getting my feet wet!")

"Congratulations, you have walked halfway across the Sahara!"

"You're our top walker—by far!"

The primary goal of the clinical trial was to evaluate the benefits of using a Fitbit to record the amount of walking done each day by the many participants in the trial. There is no question using the Fitbit encouraged Ed to set higher and higher goals. Equally important, was the regular communication Ed had with the Sargent College physical therapists at a distance, via technology. This was important as there are people with PD who can't get to a physical therapist regularly because of the expense or transportation difficulties. For Ed exercise *is* key. But, even more than that, the clinical trial showed how healing—not curing but *healing*—is about relationships. Healing, as in feeling more whole, happier, more motivated, more connected with others, with life, ideals, hopes, possibilities.

This study was really about more than just walking. It was truly about stepping out—as if out ahead of the PD symptoms, both physical and psychological. Stepping out of the worries and the isolation PD can impose on one. Ed clearly felt useful and needed. I was almost jealous of his easy rapport with those young ladies, who were always happy to see him when we went to Boston for the in-person check-ins. Yup, no question about it, I married a charmer!

Ed felt let down when that clinical trial ended, though he kept in touch with one of the therapists for awhile afterwards. But he hasn't stopped walking, though it's more like two or three miles a day, even when it's raining or the roads are icy. If too inclement, he'll do his "gerbil walk" as it calls it, round and round the basement in big circles.

I felt sad and somewhat let down myself when the clinical trial ended, as though we'd left some good-energy athletes' club where everyone is dressed in trim, sporty clothes and bouncy sneakers, all gung-ho.

Then we met John Pepper.

Right here, however, I need to express my admiration for the physical therapists of today; it has grown by leaps and bounds. My niece, Diana, whom we see maybe once a year as she lives in Wyoming, is always accessible by email, always ready to try to help figure out a way to get through a neurological thicket, or around a stumbling block, an ache, a pain.

I'm awed by the scope of understanding of physical therapists, not only of how bones, muscles and nerves interact –the harmonious and healing relationships we can rediscover or create within our bodies—but, even more, their intuitive sense of how to help patients find or reconnect with their own deep body understanding.

When Ed returns home from his physical therapy sessions he brings the feel of deepened and expanded breath, and pleasure, the pleasure of doing movements carefully, fully. The movements put him back rightly into his body, even if only for half an hour. These physical therapists offer a kind of refitting.

Physical therapy shows up close how *any* form of movement or exercise can become far more than mere physical competence. Deliberate movement can take us into subtle, spiritual dimensions that are the other half of the physical dimensions we're primarily aware of—in short into mind-body-spirit connections. My interest in this topic, stemming from the need when younger to find other ways of hearing than physical ears, led me to Matthew Sanford. He is the author of *Waking, A Memoir of Trauma and Transcendence,* and the founder of the organization, Mind-Body Solutions.

Matthew was 13 when he was in a car accident that killed his father and sister and left him paralyzed from the chest down and confined to a wheelchair. (His mother and older brother, who were also in the accident, survived, physically intact.) He struggled to rebuild his life and to enter into a new relationship with his body, even to the point of thinking that if his legs were useless, perhaps he should have them removed. Luckily his mother talked him out of that. Twelve years after the accident, Matthew met the yoga teacher who led him to what he eloquently refers to as "the body's commitment to living," no matter our age or what has happened or is happening to our physical bodies. Here's one of his descriptions:

*When yogic instruction rekindled feeling of energetic sensation within my mind-body relationship, it felt like settling into a warm bath—the relief, the feeling of nourishment, the calm and quieting reference. I grew in dimension as my **entire** body began whispering to me once again, albeit in a more eloquent voice.*

Ed hasn't, yet, been drawn to yoga. He did tai chi for a few years but the teacher he liked lived too far away. Then we discovered Dance for Parkinson's and felt an instant connection with it, the instructor, and the class. It deserves a chapter by itself.

To return to walking and to John Pepper...
I can't remember when we first heard of John and his book, *Reverse Parkinson's Disease!* Pepper, is ten years older than us, lives in South Africa and has been traveling the world for several years giving talks and demonstrations on his discoveries about PD, having had PD himself for over 50 years. He offers presentations and will coach others with PD in walking wherever folks have heard of him by way of word of mouth, or the internet, or his book.

Pepper's story is so compelling that Norman Doidge devotes an entire chapter to it in his book, *The Brain's Way of Healing Remarkable Discoveries and Recoveries from the Frontiers of Neuroplasticity,* published in 2015. There's no question in my mind this is an extremely important chapter in the history and treatment of PD. As Doidge says, Pepper is, through his discoveries, claiming there are neuroplastic ways to manage PD symptoms, stop their progress and in some cases reverse them. These neuroplastic "ways" depend on *conscious movement*, beginning with everyday walking. This means being fully aware of how one is walking as one is walking. Merely walking fast or walking a lot every day (as Ed did in the clinical trial) isn't central to Pepper's treatment. In fact, Pepper advises walking sessions of only 20 minutes three or four times a week. Pepper urges one to be consistently and constantly attentive to many things: how one stands and carries oneself, how one puts one's weight down on the feet, and more. The thesis, as I understand it, is that, when one part of the brain isn't operating, another part or other parts of the brain can take on the tasks of the non-operating part.

I was quite excited when I first heard about John's book, then, later, when we met him and his wife at a PD convention in Oregon in 2016. As I saw it he was taking the "use it or loose it" mantra several steps further and much deeper. I also felt, as I read about Pepper's path, "Ed's already doing a lot of this—he's on the right track!"

When we met Pepper in person, he promptly took the cane out of Ed's hand and handed it to me. Then he took hold of Ed's arm and walked away with him the full length of the large room we were in, and back again. I could see he was talking to Ed intently as they walked, coaching and guiding him. And I saw as they walked that Ed was upright in a way he hadn't been upright for years. There was a briskness and a vigor to his step, and no shuffling. Most stunning of all, Ed right arm was swinging, in keeping with his steps for the first time since he'd been diagnosed! My heart rose up into my throat. Had we found a way to move out beyond the shrinking, contracting, restricting walls of PD?

Pepper's excitement, enthusiasm and evident eagerness to share his discoveries were wonderful. We were on hugging terms by the time we said goodbye to him and his wife after that first meeting. The fact that Pepper wasn't invited to speak at the PD convention puzzled me, however. I'd scanned the convention program when we first arrived expecting to see his name listed there but there was no sign of it. Pepper had mentioned in his book, that the medical community in South Africa hadn't welcomed him, had even questioned whether he really has PD. I knew from his book he was able to go off medications because of practicing conscious movement and was very impressed by that. (I don't know if that is still the case.) But for others we knew with PD, that, in itself, seemed to be reason not to get involved with him. Either they didn't quite believe him, or his recommendations didn't work for them, or they were reluctant to turn their back on medications they were finding helpful.

"The medical and drug industries have *lots* of money invested in PD,"' Pepper's wife told me as we chatted while our husbands walked boldly up and down the conference hall in September of 2016. Was she implying the medical community didn't want to recognize or give any credit or space to Pepper's discoveries because those discoveries, in their simplicity and directness, might take the dollars away from them? That was a troubling thought. I didn't get to talk further or deeper with the Peppers about this because we were with them so briefly. In addition, other personal events prevented us from keeping in touch with them or seeing them again.

My own understanding is that Pepper is pointing at the importance of how one responds to PD. I don't just mean this in the usual outer sense of: are you finding the medical information you need to understand what's going on? Are you getting the best professional advice? How are the medications affecting you? Do you have a good support team? I am sure John would agree all of these are important. But, to my ear, his central message is loud and clear: how one thinks *is* the key to how one lives with PD. As John states at the start of his book,

There is no limit to what our minds and bodies are capable of achieving, if we want something badly enough.

John's "wanting" led him not only to his thoughtful rendering of conscious walking but to many other things he believes one needs to be aware of and responding to as a curious and on-going learner, not merely a patient. A quick glance at the table of contents in his book lists some of these other things: diet, stress management, attitude adjustment, mental stimulation, the effects of medications. John told us in person that when he concentrates on the things that hinder him (or others with PD) such as the freezing of gait, he's able to overcome many problems.

I don't take John's determined and self-aware stance to simply mean an alert and positive mind can find ways to figure out, manage, or move beyond every PD symptom, though, according to his book, he's done amazingly well. I believe there is more to John's success than mind over matter. Could it be that the *wanting something badly* he refers to, which motivates and activates him, is a power in itself? A power that not only focuses one's attention helping one to probe the physical situation at hand, but draws the energy of intention right into the physical body. An energy as powerful as dopamine!

To take a few steps down another path, which I think is related to the one we're on here, there's an interesting study described in another book, *Brain Storms :The Race To Unlock The Mysteries of Parkinson's Disease,* by Jon Palfreman (which I quoted from at the start of the first chapter) where PD patients in a clinical trial who were given a placebo rather than a medication, responded positively. As Palfreman wrote,

This [the result of the clinical trial] *leads to a striking conclusion. While the medicines may be fake, the placebo responses going on in our brains must be real, mediated by actual neurotransmitters.*

And, in the next paragraph,

Dopamine is known to regulate reward-seeking and novelty-seeking behaviors. So it's not hard to imagine how a dopamine-mediated placebo effect might trigger relief from pain in a healthy patient. But in Parkinson's it can't be that simple. Parkinson's is a disease defined by dopamine depletion. When symptoms first appear, perhaps 70 percent of the dopamine neurons in the substantia nigra (and an even higher proportion of the connections to the striatum) are already gone. Given this major loss, where does the brain find enough dopamine to modulate a placebo effect strong enough to cause major symptomatic improvement that can persist for years?

When I read that I thought of Pepper and wondered if the hope accompanying the *wanting* that impels a person to sign up in a clinical trail, could be likened to John's *wanting*. Maybe not as self-aware and self-motivated a wanting as John's which others may find hard to hold to or measure up to, but nevertheless a deeply valid wanting. Again, a power, an energy as powerful as dopamine. Perhaps this *wanting* could be called a spiritual or soul force that is somewhere deep within us always, similar to what Matthew Sanford, in his physical paralysis, called *the body's commitment to living*. A soul commitment to the very essence of Life.

While I admire Pepper and the PD path he is on I don't agree with his use of the word "reversing" in the title of his book. "Reversing Parkinson's" makes it sound as though one can return to the condition one was in before one was diagnosed with PD. John admits he still has many of the symptoms of PD but he is in charge of his life. That seems to be his message to the world. I wouldn't say Ed is exactly in charge of his life. (Nor am I for that matter!) How can one be in charge of the many unknowns, the many waves of all sizes from all directions that come with PD? Again and again I have seen Ed step out when he is exhausted, I have seen him swim out to meet or brace himself to meet the wave that is coming at him. I can hear his *wanting* to be a part of life, even when he has his off times and may not look altogether there physically. In this Ed, the patient, is marvelously, consistently patient, reminding me often of words from Father Thomas Keating:

"This constant starting over {every day} with patience, calm, and acceptance trains us for the whole of life."

Dancing

Something incredibly beautiful happened in our Dance for Parkinson's class today.

The whole class was sitting in a circle, and Fritha, our instructor, explained that she would do a movement and we were to mirror what she did for a few minutes. Then she would pass the role of leader on to the person on her left, and all of us would mirror whatever movements that person made. When that person had completed her movements and had seen them reflected back to her, she, in turn, would pass the leadership role to the person on her left. And so on, around the circle, the varying movements would flow, giving each dancer a chance to add his or her personal story, joke or commentary to whatever beat and mood Fritha had chosen.

We have done this many times, so we are all—there are 14 in the class right now—comfortable with this form of sharing. We are also more or less familiar with each other's bodily vocabularies: Chris with her defiant, almost military arm movements, James turning his extreme tremor again and again into a very particular kind of air weaving, Nancy, our eldest at 80, making gentle nest-building shapes with her hands, then blowing them out over all of us like rainbow bubbles.

Fritha chose a slow waltz-like piece that fit the mood of the cool misty-moisty spring day outside. What she started was in her very own Fritha vocabulary, done primarily from the waist up (some in the class can't stand easily) with big, generous, arm, elbow and hand movements that sometimes make me think of windows closing, then opening, closing, then opening wider and wider. Many of Fritha's dances echo the constrictive, narrowing, closing-in nature of PD and the corresponding effort to open, reopen, stay open, let in space and deepened breath and escape tight, rigid, habitual patterns.

Joan, to Fritha's left, went from window closing and opening into gentle arm gestures, first on one side, then the other, back and forth. It was as though we'd slipped out through our windows and were now in our canoes, paddling downstream. Then the paddling became pointing—an exclaiming over this and that on the shore, including each other, or at

49

stars overhead, or clouds in the sky.

Suzie, taking the lead from Joan, shifted our movements seamlessly from arms and hands to legs and feet. Putting our hands on our hips, we pointed with our toes, bumped the floor with our heels to the count of four, drew circles with both feet from small into bigger and bigger.

Then Suzie indicated with a slide of her left foot in Max's direction it was his turn to lead.

Max and his wife Wendy joined the class recently. They fit right in. We had learned that Wendy has always loved country dancing, that they have two grown sons, and that Max has not only PD, but also Lewy body dementia. When I heard that, I was reminded of a heart-rending personal account by a man with the same vicious combination of conditions. I wept through his book some years ago and was ashamed to feel relief that Ed hadn't been dealt that double whammy. (That account is *Life in the Balance: A Physician's Memoir of Life, Love and Loss with Parkinson's and Dementia*, by Thomas Graboys MD, with Peter Zheutlin.)

Now with word retrieval, confusion and forgetfulness starting to nag at Ed, I feel how pointless such comparisons are. It's not that we're lucky, or luckier than others—though on the outside that may indeed be the case. It's that when your heart is being broken open by life, there can be moments when you may feel your breaking merging with the breaking others are experiencing. It's as when waves, from various directions, created by different disturbances, meet and become one within a river or on the surface of a body of water. One glance at the face of another, or others, and you know what they are feeling. Their feeling washes over and into you, becoming yours, too.

Active empathy—which seems to be several notches up from mere sympathy—doesn't pause for even a second to dwell on self-protection or self-preservation. It is nonjudgmental and nondiscriminatory. It simply flows with the other, or others, offering acceptance and support. When filled with it, I've felt myself able to offer care in ways I didn't realize I was capable of offering. Later, when, so to speak, the tide of empathy has receded and I again see the person or situation as if at a distance, I may not be ready to hand that person the coat off my back, but I'm aware that my perception of the person or situation has been altered forever.

This empathy is what I experienced in the few minutes when Max was leading the mirroring activity in our dance class. Until then, he and Wendy were the newcomers. I'd chatted several times with Wendy but had made little to no effort to connect with Max. To describe him a bit: He's tall, thin and aloof. He has a pronounced PD tremor in his left hand. That hand can flutter frantically like a leaf on a tree limb being whipped this way and that by the wind. He also has a pronounced, flat, expressionless PD mask and hardly ever speaks. So, in class, everyone's communications with this couple tend to be with Wendy, not with him. For the most part Max simply stands, or sits, beside his wife while you're talking with her. You have no idea whether he's listening to what's being said, though there can be a watchful look in his brown eyes.

Today, however, when asked to lead, Max seemed to understood perfectly. I'd never seen such decisive movements from him. He stood, turned, faced his wife and slowly began slapping both arms with his hands without taking his eyes off her face. She mirrored back what he was doing. The rest of us who could stand jumped up, trying to follow along, but that was hard because he was now standing sideways. Wendy had turned sideways also, to face him, so you couldn't get the all of what they were doing. It looked as though they were having a very private, very intimate conversation. To my eyes it was as though this taciturn man, who must now be a shadow of his former self, had suddenly reclaimed his voice in movement.

Within seconds the tremor in his hand calmed and the slapping hand movements morphed into gentle, fluid, giving gestures. Wendy accepted whatever Max was giving her and turned—flushed and wide-eyed-- to face the rest of the class, to continue the mirroring dance. Max also turned away from her, back to us, back into the tight place we've known him to inhabit, his left hand again fluttering wildly. Whether we knew it or not, I believe we all had, briefly, seen Max—not the man with PD and Lewy body dementia, but Max, the man Wendy had married, the man she knew long before they joined our class.

There have been other moments like this in our dance class. They come and go as quickly as a leap or a twirl. Some are deep, even dark, while others are high, light, silly. You can feel something has changed and later wonder, "What was it?" Perhaps it felt as though the incessant wind ceased for a time and we all just bobbed about happily on the surface of a blue-green ocean.

At times I'm moved almost to tears by the eloquence, the grace and honesty of a gesture, a facial expression, a meditatively slow or a happy-quick turn. Fritha's class provides an opportunity for everybody present—whether with or without PD-- to have his or her say in the midst of daily frustrations surrounding ordinary mobility and caregiving. And there can be a lot that needs to be expressed! Steve can, at the start of class, look so heavy, so burdened. Liz can, also at the start, seem downright depressed. Sometimes I wonder if the dancers are aware how much their bodies are saying, or trying to say. Is it that music and dance give us opportunities to step out of or beyond self-consciousness into some lovely spaciousness where we are beyond pretension? Where we are truly ourselves?

I have to give Fritha the credit she deserves for making the incredibly beautiful moments possible. She was a performing dancer, then had her own dance troupe, then later trained in Dance for Parkinson's at the Mark Morris Dance Company in Brooklyn, New York with by David Lowenthal. We know that being in her class is *not* like being in a ballroom dancing class. We are not learning to waltz, hip-hop, rhumba and cha-cha, though there may be elements of every kind of dancing Fritha ever did woven into her classes. Every sequence of steps she makes up and leads us through has its own flicker, ripple and shimmer. She shows us how to be soaring birds, buzzing bees, stretching trees, sun-kissing plants, self-contained turtles. She takes us beyond any worry as to how stiff, clumsy, awkward or plain ridiculous we might feel or look. *Every* try counts. She is always there offering her smile of support, without any coddling, always there with her reassuring, "Any questions?" should we feel overly challenged or confused as to exactly what we're doing. I've never seen her become impatient when we ask her to repeat a sequence over and over and over. Plain, bold, beautiful and outrageous dancers and socks: all are welcome. I specially love how, after her demonstration and after the questions have been answered and the hesitations have been met, Fritha says, "Here we go!" as she jumps up to turn the music on.

Fritha's youth is a tonic for this slowed-down gaggle of seniors, and so is the youth of Fritha's volunteer assistant, Suzie, who provides water and snacks during our break and, when dancing, moves like a sheep-herding dog among us, nudging us this way and that.

And my Ed? Where is he in all this? We are nearly always partners, sitting side by side or facing one another when doing mirroring and

52

improvisational dances. After days and nights of living side by side, it's good to look directly, intentionally, at my other half. To move together, to meet each other's eyes, to smile or wink, to express befuddlement at the complexity of a foot pattern Fritha is introducing.

"How does that go?" Ed's face asks.

"I have no idea," I reply with a shrug.

Seconds later, Fritha picks up on our puzzlement. We can't bluff. She clarifies, and not just once, but three times. We imitate her movements, often wondering later why it's so hard to recall exactly how these movements go. Are we more in our heads than our bodies? Do our bodies have their own ways of remembering? I *want* these movements to become habits, the way memorized poems are often friends in dark or difficult moments.

Every now and then in class I find myself across the room from Ed. Suddenly I'm seeing him as I see our fellow dancers with PD. This little bit of separation and distance can be jarring, in the same way that catching that glimpse of us in a store window while crossing the street was jarring. Now I am being forced to see the wear and tear, the daily advance of PD. I see Ed's thinness, the hunch of his shoulders, the lack of clear articulation by his feet, his shuffle and the lines of fatigue. I also see his uncertainties. Can he do it? Is he doing it right? Can he summon the energy to get through it? The uncertainties hurt the most. Active empathy stirs in me, reaches out across the space to him. All I know is that I want the music to come like a breaking wave, wash over us all, wash away the worries and fears in all of us, carry us on in this kaleidoscope of bright, gay movements.

And it does!

Again and again!

Thank you, Fritha!

It Is As It Is

Every other Friday I go to my caregivers' support group meeting. Each meeting is different, has its own flavor, is created not only by who can make it that day, but by the ebb and flow of seasons. By seasons I don't just mean the seasons of the year, although we're all quite aware of those, but the seasons of aging—of wondering now and then if we're losing our marbles, of having to figure out how to manage financial resources or find medical or nursing assistance—and the seasons of loss and of grieving. Some still in the vale of grieving continue to come for a while after the one they've been caring for has passed over.

Anne, our wise and steady facilitator, lost her husband 15 years ago, suddenly, in his mid fifties. She keeps an eye on the clock, keeps things moving along, makes sure everyone's heard while providing sympathetic and gritty commentary and comfort. She listens behind and between our words and draws attention to themes that come, go, and pop up yet again like simmering fevers. Helplessness, impatience, frustration and loneliness seem to be the primary fevers. Relief comes in recognizing and acknowledging them as Anne identifies them both at the start of the meeting, then again at the end, skillfully, gently. And sometimes her sweet labradoodle comes with her and checks in with us too, going from person to person, licking an elbow here, nudging a leg there.

Christine is Anne's "other hand." The warmth of their friendship is the fire around which we gather. Christine is a retired nurse practitioner who, again and again, provides information and helpful insight into medical issues. Her husband also has PD. Her familiarity with the health-care system and insurance issues, both local and statewide, is extremely reassuring. There are often stories of exhausted caregivers overwhelmed by confusing paperwork, snappish secretaries, complex medical procedures. The linear everyday world seems to have a ridiculous number of regulations about what you're supposed to do when someone you love is either slipping-sliding or zigzagging his or her way out into the other world. It's as though everything depends on a signature on a piece of paper from years ago--and where the heck *is* that paper? As though X years of marriage are suddenly being reduced to the question,

"Is this *really* what he or she wants?" As though a death certificate is the only way you can prove someone has died. Isn't death evident just by looking in a face? By that I mean not only the face of the one who has passed over but the face of the caregiver who is still here.

Christine pulled me into this group shortly after it started, though Ed and I aren't members of the church where it meets and most in the caregivers' group are. We do occasionally attend the services there and always feel welcome. I'm especially grateful for the very definite presence of faith in our meetings: faith in the power and grace of listening, and faith in the belief that we not only hold one another when listening but are held by God. This listening calls forth deep honesty. There's no scale of 1 to 10 in terms of who's got the heaviest load, is most in need or is saying things most powerfully, though there are moments when I sense the grief of another as though it's mine, too. I am able to forget myself and our (Ed's and my) situation when listening in this way. I also believe God has His own staff of Caregivers. Caregivers who look after caregivers. And when we meet there are quite a few invisible Others who join us.

Almost every time we meet I sense how healing (I am not speaking here of curing; more on this elsewhere) lies in relationships—in finding, making and maintaining them, in connecting and knowing one is not alone. And these relationships spring out of mutual respect, trust and honesty, the deep honesty mentioned earlier. It's deep because this honesty comes from deep down, and it takes courage to reach down and pull it up and out for others to see and examine. When I hear and witness this honesty coming from others, I want to be equally honest in my own speaking. It feels sacrilegious not to try to honor this spirit. If I'm not up to that or can't bring myself to it, it seems better to say nothing.

Sometimes the honesty of this group asks me to think, in turn, about honesty in my everyday life. How honest should I be with colleagues, friends, family, even Ed? There are times when I frankly don't feel like going into the depths as someone looks me in the eyes and asks, "How *are* you?" It's better right then not to go there because I might get stuck there, and it's important—both for Ed and me—that we keep going, keep moving.

I've also pondered how what we think of as honesty can belittle or discourage rather than clear out, build up, strengthen. Raw honesty can wound, can be more about the speaker than the one being spoken to. Tactful honesty holds the self in check. I often hear this tactful honesty when Anne shares her observations:

"Mariam, from what I'm hearing I'm wondering if *you* need help." she'll say. Rather than what might have popped out of my mouth, "Mariam, stop trying to do *everything* for Nancy!"

I've noticed too how the truth may sting at moments but also empower. Along the same line, the truth that's being uttered may be directed at someone else, yet I can hear it as though it's being said to me! This happened recently when Tom was advising Jen about the advance of dementia in her husband, and how that would be limiting his physical mobility more and more.

Jen nodded. She was already experiencing this contraction, was aware her husband's world—and therefore hers too—was pulling backward, inward, shrinking.

"Travel when you can," Tom told her. "Make memories when you can."

I heard those words and knew he was right. Later, that night, Ed and I talked about a "manageable" trip to Florida. We'd been a bit unnerved the year before after we'd made plans to live out a long-time dream to go to Alaska and had to cancel the whole trip when Ed had a close call. (Which I speak of in another chapter.) Alaska was suddenly *very* far from home. Did we want to have another close call way up there among strangers while looking at polar bears?

I'm humbled and often moved beyond words by the honesty in this caregivers' group. The feelings expressed are real, and I've felt at moments as though I'm looking at open wounds. Most speak without tears, though you know right away when tears are close to the surface. And newcomers sometimes weep during their first visit and are clearly embarrassed to find themselves crying. I understand those tears. They're tears of relief. Relief at finding one's self in a safe place and being able to put into words what was weighing on one.

There's a dignity to everyone. Sometimes you know a person is holding back as though not wanting to drag others down. You might say it's a Yankee trait; my father certainly had it. I see it in Ed, too, and I respect it. Whether it stems from not wanting to bother others, feeling basically that one's problems are one's own to sort out, or feeling that to complain is to sound ungrateful, I'm not sure. This reserve of something (Hope? Faith? Gratitude?) seems good and necessary to me. This hesitation when being honest, this reluctance to go too far—is this related to the presence of our better selves, our guardian angel?

Today Gail's load is unusually heavy. Her husband is backing away, week by week, day by day, into forgetfulness, unresponsiveness. She describes him sitting in his chair, motionless, staring at nothing and nobody. He was a train engineer. She shows me a photo of his toy trains —shiny reminders of when the engine *in* him was still running at full throttle.

Ona's husband, who fell and had a severe brain injury told her recently the bathroom "moved." We all laugh when we hear that and, briefly, venture into fantasy. How does a bathroom move? Can it shake itself, dance, inch its way elsewhere in the house?

Ona explains her understanding of her husband's comment: The washing machine and drier are behind the door to the bathroom. There was too much laundry in the drier and it spilled out, closing the bathroom door. So that was the movement her husband heard and saw.

Peggy then describes one of her husband's obsessions: shaving. After he's shaved in the morning he's convinced he hasn't. This happens several times a day. Peggy keeps on reminding him to feel the smoothness of his own cheeks.

Then Gail has a harrowing tale to tell about an insurance mix-up. She describes frantic calls to connect with her insurance agent and not being able to get beyond "Press one for.... Press two for...Press three for...." with no amount of pressing yielding any results.

Finally she was able to reach someone who agreed to keep an eye on her husband. She drove for over an hour to the insurance company, had to wait another three hours—and the young man she was lucky enough to talk with cleared it up in 15 minutes! We all cheer.

But Gail isn't done. Two days later, she received a notice that her Medicare benefits had been stopped. The wild phoning started up again, until that, too, was resolved.

We clap again, but this second cheer is quite a bit more restrained.

"I'm worn out by it all," Gail declares. "It's an emotional roller coaster."

She *does* look worn out. I want to reach out and touch her, but I don't. It feels as though she needs the being heard far more than any hugging.

I do hug Lou, though. She is sitting across from me and barely looks up. She has a quick, radiant smile—but no smile today. Her eyes are downcast (yes, there is such a thing as downcast eyes—very definitely.) I am glad when Anne says, ever so kindly, "And Lou…?" when it is Lou's turn during check-in.

Lou is dealing with two at once: her dad who had a stroke and her partner who has stomach cancer. Her candle is burning at both ends. When she comes over to me at the end of the meeting to ask about a book on trees I'd mentioned, I catch her up in a hug. She brightens as we share tree stories.

How easy I have it, by comparison, with Ed! The waves we're dealing with are much smaller. It may not always be this way but, for now, I am grateful; grateful for these glimpses into the lives and loves of others.

As might be expected from the number of senior men versus senior women in the population today, there are more women than men in our group. Ed has said for sometime that I will very likely outlive him. And my response is, "How can you be so sure? As it is now—with PD slowing you down—I'm often a couple of steps ahead of you" -- meaning I just might decide to go first! I could get the breakfast table ready in advance of his arrival, with some excellent pecan granola. Then to heck from then on with the need for prunes, like turtles, atop the tasty, golden, nutty mix. Is there such a thing as constipation in Heaven?

Considering the statistics, who was it that first said women are the weaker sex?

I think of that often when I go to the YMCA Monday mornings to swim and the seniors are having their social hour together at the tables set up in the hallway. So many white-haired ladies babbling together, while a single silent guy or two stand over there on the fringes of it all.

It's the same in the caregivers group: two men, seven to nine women.

My father outlived my mother by 12 years, but he was devastated by her death. All the health issues of his own that he'd ignored because his focus was entirely on her monumental health issues suddenly caught up with him. He was really knocked out for awhile. It turned out he even had Lyme disease and hadn't known it.

When his health improved, he began to chafe at our hovering over him. He was 85 then and still amazingly mobile (though with some vision difficulties.)   He approached a dear friend, who had also been a nurse to my mother, asking for help with shopping and cooking. Marge was delighted to be of assistance.

Soon my father was asking Marge to stay and eat the meals she'd prepared with him. Then he, as she was uncomfortable driving in the dark, suggested she stay the night. After all, there were extra rooms and beds in the house.

I remember the Columbus Day weekend Ed and I, and my brother and his wife also, were visiting with my father. Ed and I arrived first, and the minute I stepped into the kitchen I knew something was different. The atmosphere was lighter, brighter. My father greeted us with surprising enthusiasm.

"I want to show you some towels upstairs in your mother's bathroom," he told me

Towels in my mother's bathroom? Baffled, I followed him upstairs into the bathroom.

"The most wonderful thing happened," he said closing the door.

I nodded for him to go on.

"Last night," he explained, "I was reading in bed and fell asleep with the bedside light on..."

Another nod to indicate I had heard and was following his story.

"And someone came in and turned the light off ..."

He paused for a fraction of a second.

"...and hugged me!" he hurried on. Then in a rush, "It was the most wonderful thing to be hugged!"

I'd known about Marge preparing meals for him, but hadn't known that had advanced to sharing meals with him and staying the night. But I understood instantly from his words and his excited boyish tone that they had moved swiftly from mere friendship into romance.

" I *don't* plan to marry her!" my father insisted as he saw the light of comprehension on my face. "I love your mother forever!"

"Daddy," I said, hugging him, "I'm *so* glad you have a companion!" I *was* glad. *So* glad.

"A companion?" he stepped back as though offended. "I'm *not* talking about a mere companion. What will people think? What do *you* think?"

"This is wonderful!" I said. "Many people who aren't married live together..."

He still looked offended, as though I hadn't really heard him.

It was evident right then he must have been starved for physical contact—indeed, for sex—during the years he'd taken care of my mother. And how thrilled he was he'd found it.

And how conflicted, too.

"People are going to say I have a mistress. "Right then he looked—upright and principled man he was—quite dismayed.

I almost laughed. A mistress? The word sounded so old-fashioned. But I'm glad I didn't laugh, because the matter was obviously of great import to him.

"Daddy, "I repeated my observation "lots of people who aren't married live together these days."

I saw from his face that he still didn't think I was getting it.

We went back downstairs. Marge wasn't around right then, I'm sure she knew he was planning to tell us about them. A short while later, when my brother and sister-in-law arrived, my father took my brother upstairs to our mother's bathroom to look at the towels and when they came back down my father was beaming.

Later I learned my brother had given our dad the "right" response: "That's great, Daddy! Now I don't have to worry about you!" No talk about couples who aren't married living together and that being okay. He wanted us to know he wouldn't remarry (he didn't) and he wanted our okay. Not because it was accepted behavior in modern times, but because he was doing something that was good for us as well as for him.

This is not to say that my father didn't love Marge. I know he did. Marge moved in with him soon afterwards and added 10 years to his life. My father told me quite a few times how wonderful it was that they had many of the same memories – of the Depression and the World War II years—and knew so many of the same stories, authors, actors and songs. We are forever grateful to Marge for her love for him and her expert care, especially during the last four years when he was shadowed by dementia.

Shortly after Marge moved in, my father called up an English cousin of my mother's to get the okay from her, too. Eliza, whom my father and I had long ago nicknamed "The rear admiral" because of her perfunctory replies to just about everything, responded pretty much this way to my father's cohabitation:

"Women know how to manage when they lose a man. They are *not*, by a long shot, the weaker sex. However…" potent pause here, "…when a man looses a woman, he doesn't know how to manage. He needs a woman."

My father laughed at that and agreed. There had been no mention of him having a mistress.

The comment from the rear admiral drifts in and out of my mind every now and then during our caregivers' support group meetings. It also reminds me right then, as I look across the table at Elaine, who lost her husband recently and still looks wiped-out, that life goes on. One never knows what new chapters may unfold.

I was a little taken back by Darrel's evident need when he first joined the group, the need to talk and talk. The family members he is caring for, through phone conversations, snail mail and email, are at a distance. How can you help from a distance without feeling rather helpless?

Some of the women knit during our time together and it has looked to me, when Darrel is speaking, as though they become yet more deeply involved in what they are doing. As if, through their regular, rhythmic hand movements they are knitting him over the miles into the situations he's describing.

When he starts talking I remind myself of the Swedish proverb, "*A sorrow shared is halved…*"

And sometimes—at the end of our hour—when he has a poem he wants to read aloud the second half of the saying washes, briefly, over us all, "*A joy shared is doubled.*"

Today Tom, whose wife has Alzheimer's, is sounding less overwhelmed than two weeks ago.

"I'm beginning to realize Dottie is *never* going to be my Dottie again," he says.

His curly gray hair is more tousled than usual. His brown eyes are moist. He haltingly describes his most recent communication – which evidently doesn't feel to him like real communication--with Dottie. She speaks, she kind-of answers, but there's no definite sign of a thread sewing words and shared meanings together. Tom is slowly giving up hope the thread is going to reemerge. What complicates things is the fact that the new health care person coming in to help Tom dress, feed and assist Dottie, has called forth a cheerful response from Dottie.

"Why does this person, a stranger in our house, get a nicer greeting from Dottie than me?" Tom asks.

"Dottie always liked meeting new people," Kathy offers.

"I remember her greeting visitors at church," Lou agrees.

"But she's happier to see this person, whom we didn't even know a week ago... than me." Tom's voice has dropped to a whisper.

No one knows what to say.

"...and I'm her husband of over 50 years!"

Still no one knows what to say. There's the need for the response to be as truthful as the offering is raw hearted.

I can *feel* what he's saying. I know I would feel the same if Ed behaved this way.

"I hear you..." Ona finally says. "I really do. *But...*"

Ona looks across the table at Tom full face, pausing a second as though weighing her words, "...Tom... it is as it is."

The way she says it is both tough, as in "Hitch up your pants, pull up your chin," and tender. *So* tender. We can't help but feel the truth of her words because they are really addressed not only to Tom but to every single one of us.

Life is as it is!

Amen!

Sleeping Later

Ed is sleeping later in the morning.

He's often annoyed and embarrassed by this, is not willing to acknowledge the energy that's missing, that's been taken away. And now getting up has become a chore. Even walking to the bathroom before the medication has taken effect is a chore. His gait freezes up, and he lurches from bedpost to doorway to bookshelf to bathroom.

I love him for his unwillingness to let go of the expectation that the energy *is* there, inside him still, intact, healthy, present, waiting to be drawn upon. And there *is* some of that energy—after all, something does get him up, even as it gets me up. But there are also the moments when I fear he's expecting too much, is unrealistic, unnecessarily hard on himself. I worry this ebbing away will take from the light that keeps him getting up and going.

How much to do—to will—and how much to let go, with the hope and expectation something else, something powerful, will come, lift one up, move one into the wonderful, utterly amazing commandment Christ gave the physically handicapped man, "*Take up thy bed and walk...*" (John 5:8) Something powerful from without, yet moving within, into, through, and out of the body into motion. Something moving into a deep knowing, "I can do this myself, I can bring the light and strength of my own incarnation into this very task, *this* moment."

(Yup, not just get up, wake up, but take up the whole damn bed, bed frame, mattress, blanket, sheets, pillows and all, and walk! I sometimes wonder what sort of bed the man with palsy had.)

Holding on and letting go, *that* is what incarnation is about in these later, senior years, with or without PD.

Ed is sleeping later in the morning.

Sometimes here, in my study, a room away from our bedroom, I can hear his breathing. It's heavy, not exactly labored, but heavy and heavier. He needs new breath to fill himself, his whole body. And an entire body is pretty big when you stop to think about it: not just lungs, not just mouth, nose, heart, not just brain, but *everything*, all the way down to the pads on the toes we stand on.

I am so glad—so relieved—when he can sleep pretty much straight through the night. There are occasions when he can't get there, and I find him sitting despondently in his office, trying to read a book, or answer an email, or he's switching the TV from channel to channel. He has found some interesting stories in those late late TV rambles. Yet those usually are the times when he winds up resorting to taking "a little bit"—not even half of a half—of an over-the-counter sleeping pill, a baby blue pill that knocks him out. When he takes the little bit he does sleep later the next morning—much later—and when he comes out of this later sleep he says he feels disconnected, drugged, a bit of a zombie. I, too, prefer it when his waking flows naturally from night into dawn into day into today—not some disconnected jumble of time. How funny and curious that that "little bit" that anybody can get at the drugstore should affect him so powerfully, he who has to take an expensive cocktail of PD meds faithfully, daily, every three hours.

Ed is sleeping later in the morning.

His is the breathing of one who is far away, further away than he was a year ago, certainly farther away than 10 years ago. Perhaps he's being called out elsewhere night by night, onto another planet, another land. What's he doing out there? Planning the building of another house? Getting to know another country—picking one where he might move when this house is beyond repair? Yes, he goes out far at night, yet he's also anchored here. His hand reaches for me when I slip into bed. "Just checking," says that hand. His breath is becoming breath sent from afar, a machine slowing down dramatically, moving back into first gear, moving out of the steady hum of second or third gear.

One morning, a little while ago, I heard from where I was downstairs, not his breathing in sleep but another strange, fitful, rattling sound. Was he calling for help? I raced up the stairs and found him seated on the edge of the bed. There was orange stuff on his face, on the bed and on the floor. He was choking—was trying to throw-up medication stuck in his throat. I grabbed him by the shoulders to shake him. Then grabbed more water for him to drink, then a waste basket, then paper towels, then orange juice. The choking subsided, he wanted to lie down again but was afraid. So I pulled the rocker over by the bed and he moved to that to be upright.

In that moment as I sat beside him I felt how close the other side is—how it is right there in the still brightness of the early spring morning—how friends and family I could not make out with my usual every-day usual eyes were standing with us. And Ed could just slip over—how easy that could be. I felt greatly, deeply, reassured by the realization but did not tell him about it till later as I knew—rightly—he might think it a bit spooky.

Ed is sleeping later.

I like knowing where he is as the sun comes up: still in our bed. I like setting the table for his breakfast, pouring his cereal, putting the three prunes like turtles on top of his cereal, starting the coffee, which we both will have, splitting a grapefruit which we will share. I like feeding the dog, checking my emails, reading the lead stories in the paper, planning my day… waiting for him to come down the stairs.

There are times, though, when he sleeps later than I like and I feel the day has not only begun, it is passing—precious hours on the run.

Funny Mouth Movements

For over a year and a half Ed has had these funny mouth movements. I mean funny as in odd, out of the ordinary, unusual, new. They are amusing in a way, but also very definitely not amusing, more puzzling than amusing, an indicator that something's off, different, changing. One can call it a new PD symptom, but a symptom reflecting what? One can feel like a detective at times. Is a circuit in the brain backfiring, getting things mixed up, trying to find some other outlet?

Andrew, at Ed's charter school, noticed the funny mouth movements at about the same time I did and mentioned them to Ed. Andrew's mother, who'd had PD, had had them, so I took it that Andrew was very kindly letting Ed know of this small change in his appearance. I asked Ed then if he was aware of this and he said yes and no: yes in that his mouth felt unusually dry and he was trying to do something about that; no, in that the internal discomfort (the dryness) and his mouth's natural effort to do something about that, had translated into an external oddity.

The hope immediately reared up in me that others *not* notice it, that others *not* look carefully and then more carefully, and write Ed off as weird. I felt a fierce, protective urge, a defiant urge, too: "He's fine inside despite what you may see outside!"

What are these funny mouth movements? Actually Ed doesn't seem to be aware when his mouth is moving in this odd manner. It can look as if he's trying to figure something out, in the same way he's trying to figure out how to move easily, move as usual, when his gait freezes up, when the festination strikes. It's a kind of mouth festination, in the same way there's a foot/feet festination. Come to think of it, I'd say there's thought festination and emotional festination, too.

It can also look as though Ed is chewing an odd-sized piece of chewing gum or a too-large piece of beef. Or he's trying to get his teeth lined up properly, but they and his lips keep sliding sideways.

The medical explanation for the involuntary spastic movements that can happen to people with PD— at least one explanation—is that the number one medication for treating PD –Sinemet—has reached the

69

ultimate helpful level of dosage one's body can absorb (that level being different for each person). When one reaches this level, the helpful effects of Sinemet—calming the tremor, halting the freezing of gait—are reversed and become unhelpful effects. Chemically the balance is upset. What one has gained becomes disturbance and loss of another sort. *Dystonia* and *dyskinesia* are two medical terms used to describe the erratic facial and physical movements that can occur. They are a curious, and scary phenomenon, a reminder that one has become dependent on this medication, so dependent the tide has turned against it.

Is there a natural, inherent, sovereignty in the body itself, as within the soul, when it says, "No more! I can't take this!"? A sovereignty that can't or shouldn't be violated? In the natural order of things that would be death or even the body taking us close to death to remind us of its needs, limits and boundaries.

Our dependency on drugs is, clearly, a two-edged sword, yet I have a great deal of gratitude for these drugs, and now more than ever. It's clear the Sinemet helps Ed, enables him to function as "normally" as he could hope. Ed can feel— and I can see—when the Sinemet is wearing off, when the gas tank is going on empty. The doctor is encouraging us to get it down to a science; he tells Ed to take Sinemet every three hours and to pay attention to what, for Ed, is the best interval between doses. This need to pay close attention to what works and what doesn't—one day everything seems to be lined up yet the funny mouth movements appear making it clear things *aren't* quite lined up—is totally new to us. In the past, as with antibiotics for infections for instance, Ed took his medication on schedule and that was that.

And how lucky we are to have the resources to cover Ed's drug expenses! There are a few other drugs as well too, like foot soldiers lined up behind behind Captain Sinemet. How many people with PD, all over the world, don't know about these medications, let alone have access to them?

Sinemet: a little, round, pale yellow pill, a tiny bit of sun.

No, it's too pale to be a bit of sun. Is it organic, inorganic, natural, man-made...? The more names and terms we collect on this journey the more we realize how much we don't know.

(The two drugs in Sinemet are carbidopa and levodopa. Since writing this chapter, Ed has shifted to a new, timed-release capsule form of carbidopa and levodopa named Rytary. Sinemet is, however, the more well-known brand name of the medication. The name, Sinemet, means "without vomiting" as early dosages of levodopa caused nausea and vomiting.)

The funny mouth movements are so unlike Ed as I have always known him. Even now, over a year later, I can't get used to them, can't think of them as part of him. Should I be able to accept them or simply ignore them? I'm able to think of my fellow swimmer and friend, Mike, as Mike, not as the man who lost his legs below the knee to meningitis. Likewise, I think of my deaf friends as people rather than as Deafies. And I know all our PD friends as people who happen to have PD. In short, I see *them* first and am open to and accepting of whatever situations or conditions come with them.

But right now I see that, with Ed and our marriage, there is territory I am *not* willing to cede to PD. These funny mouth movements and what they portend are *not* a part of him as I've always known and know him. It's possible I might think of them differently if I was just meeting him and had never known him speaking freely without them. But I feel them as a threat, a threat to our ability to communicate. Though they may seem small beside the foot festinations which could lead to a fall, they feel to me like possibly the biggest wave we've encountered thus far.

Again and again PD asks—or rather invites—us to find our way into new ways of perceiving the physical human body and its many surprising and inherent abilities. Maybe these funny mouth movements aren't an aberration, maybe Ed and I are at the start of finding another language...?

71

Close Calls

It was the day after we'd returned from a PD convention in Portland, Oregon. Ed wanted to go to dance class as usual, and I needed to catch up with our snail mail, stock the refrigerator, do the laundry, and other such things, so I didn't accompany him.

About five hours after he'd left to drive the 29 or so miles to Northampton by himself, I was sitting at the kitchen table paying bills when the Jetta pulled into the driveway. I noticed from where I was sitting that he hadn't opened the garage door as he always does to drive the car in, and there was something funny about the side of the car.

I went to the back door and Ed stumbled into the house visibly shaken. He told me he had dozed off on his way, driving about 65 miles an hour. He was in the left lane when he dozed off, the car had veered to the left and the horrible sound of the guard railing tearing at the side of the car had awakened him. Startled, Ed veered to the right, then off the road over the rumble strip, coming to an abrupt stop on the grass. Minutes later a young man who had seen what had happened pulled up ahead of Ed and walked over to check on him.

Ed was very grateful for the concern and the kind manner of this man whose wife was in their car. The couple followed him to the next exit, the one we always take, and Ed drove on home safely from there. There were white scratch and tear marks on the side of the Jetta, but the damage wasn't so serious that he couldn't open the driver's door.

A few days later, when on the highway, I saw exactly where this close call had occurred. I thanked God for the guard rail. If Ed had fallen asleep just a few feet further on, where there was no guard rail, the car would very likely have tumbled into a ravine. And I thanked God no other cars, including the one carrying the young man and his wife, were close behind Ed when he veered to the right because they would surely have hit him.

In an earlier chapter I described a premonition. Curiously, when we were in Oregon for the convention I'd had a premonition of this close call. It happened when we were driving to Portland from Mt. Hood with relatives. I was in the front passenger seat beside Ben, the driver. Ed was in the back seat with his cousin, Theo. I suddenly inwardly "saw" a driver in a car fall sleep, causing the car to veer to the right. I looked at Ben. He seemed okay, but I offered to drive if he wanted a break. He said he was fine. I figured if Ben did fall asleep and veered to the right the rumble strip would wake him up. But I remained alert all the way back to Portland, making small talk with Ben, to be sure he was awake.

When Ed stumbled into the house and told me what had happened, I felt cold all over. What I'd "seen" *had* happened! This was as far as I can remember the second time in my life I'd had a wide-awake visual premonition. My other premonitions were "heard," as when I heard the word Parkinson's or saw events in dreams.

Ed wanted to know what the message was in that close call. We talked about it for several days afterwards. I thought it was pretty obvious. He'd been tired from the trip home, had not had enough sleep the night before, was going from one time zone to another, which had also thrown his medications a bit off schedule, and should no longer assume his body could make shifts of this sort. As I too am forced to admit as I age, I've taken my physical energy for granted for years. And, heck, where'd I get the idea I'm still brand new? It takes longer to get over colds, sprains, aches, pains, late nights, sleepless nights, and so on. Add to those the emotional hurts, upsets, frustrations, disappointments, which can be the cause of the sleepless nights, and so on.

But, even though Ed had been dealing with PD for eight years at that point, this close call brought the PD—unwanted reminder of physical decline—a good deal closer.

For months after this incident, Ed wasn't sure he wanted to drive to Northampton or other long distances, and I could see, or feel, him flinch when I was driving and (in his opinion) drove too close to someone's mailbox or the edge of the road. If I took what he thought was a sudden turn, it was as if the air was sucked right out of him.

The next close call occurred about six months later. I described it in the last chapter when I was in the kitchen, heard weird sounds coming from upstairs, raced up to our bedroom and found Ed choking on one of the orange pills he'd just taken. Ed was quite shaken by that experience. (Choking, in the later stages of PD, can become a problem as normal swallowing movements may be hindered or impaired.)

It was a bit different for me. As we bobbed about on the ocean of our daily lives after that experience I found what stayed with me was

74

the thought, "We simply stop breathing when we pass over." It *wasn't* a thought that scared me. There was something matter-of-fact about it. We go from breathing—which we all know is essential for being alive—to not breathing. When we stop breathing what happens to us? Where do *we* (the core, the soul that is us) go? How does it feel? Can we still see, hear, touch others even if we, apparently, can't breathe?

These may sound like aimless wonderings but I felt deeply humbled by them, as though, to speak metaphorically, I'd actually touched with my fingers the veil between breathing and not breathing, between here and there. I *could* feel the veil. It was as real to me right then as my own skin.

On a practical level, Ed asked the doctor if the orange pills, which he called the footballs because of their shape and size, could be taken some other way. We'd both heard of pills being ground up and mixed with applesauce as an easier way to get them down. The doctor responded with an emphatic "no" because the purpose of the footballs was to facilitate the slow timed-release of another medication. Grinding them into a powdery form would speed everything up. The doctor did say, though, that the footballs could be taken halved, so there was less chance of the whole pill getting stuck in Ed's throat.

I found halving the footballs in the plastic pill cutter a very decisive act. It was actually fun! Curious how a little task like that can make one feel useful.

A few months later, Ed had another close call with the orange pills. This time I was reading in the living room and heard him choking in the kitchen. The sound came from yet deeper down in Ed and was a lot harsher and more persistent.

Ed was red in the face and wobbly. The retching and coughing continued. I knew I couldn't do the Heimlich maneuver, because I'd cracked a rib a couple of weeks earlier and didn't have the strength. I got him a glass of water, then a bit of applesauce, then ice cream, thinking something smoother, cooler and more solid than water might get whatever there was of that half-a- football down his throat. But Ed gestured toward the phone.

I got out the TTY put the telephone receiver on it, dialed the TTY relay number, and asked the operator to get 911. Within a few minutes I'd typed out our address and information about Ed's condition and was told help would be on the way immediately. (For those unfamiliar with the TTY, it is a text telephone used by the deaf to communicate. Both the caller and the party being called have to use a TTY. In this instance I was talking with a relay operator who typed with me but talked directly on the phone with the police.)

Though I was told help was coming the relay operator wouldn't let me hang up. He or she obviously wanted to help monitor the situation and keep me connected till the help arrived, but Ed had walked out of the kitchen!

I left the TTY and ran into the living room and then the hall, looking for him. He shuffled out of the back bathroom and back into the kitchen. The coughing was milder and sounded much more like an irritation than an outright emergency. He nodded that he was better.

About eight minutes after I'd made the connection with 911, when the person I was typing with was still wanting to know how things were going, and my spelling was becoming sloppier and sloppier because I wanted to pay attention to Ed, not to the TTY, a local policeman and a town selectman arrived. We both remembered the selectman from the last town meeting. Mr. Manners—really his name—was all good manners. He radiated calm, steadiness and reassurance and was not at all rattled by Ed's condition. He said it looked as though the worst was over, but the ambulance was coming anyway to take Ed to the hospital to check that no part of the football was lodged in his lung.

The ambulance came, and I followed in our car. We waited in the ER for a couple of hours till the doctor could examine him and let him go. He suggested, in view of the fact that this had happened more than once, that Ed make an appointment with a specialist and take a swallowing test.

If there was a message in this close call, it was, I felt, addressed to me. I *could* use the TTY to get help—I didn't have to run out into the night for a neighbor—and help *could* come very fast—with perfectly wonderful manners! I'd witnessed those emergency calls when my dad was declining but had never been overseeing the situation all by myself. Was it a rehearsal of some sort?

I also "heard" Ed when his fourth close call occurred. I was again in the living room, and this time he called for help.

I ran out to the kitchen and found him by the sink, blood pouring from his hand. He'd been cutting wood on the band saw in the basement and the wood had slipped. At first I thought his hand had been cut by the band saw. Then, as I ran water over the cut, I saw that the saw had shattered the edge of the wood and a splinter from it had gone deep into the middle finger of his left hand.

Ed said he'd pulled the splinter out. But was there still wood in the wound? Did he need stitches? Ed thought he might. He quite literally turned green at this point and stumbled forward against the counter as if about to faint.

My instinct was to stop the blood flow as best as possible and prevent him from falling. I wrapped the finger in a wad of paper towels, then gauze pad and tape, helped him onto the sofa in the living room and got his feet up. Then water to drink, something light to eat and he dosed off for a while. The crisis had passed. But our boat continued to rock for awhile.

Ed took himself to the ER the next afternoon. More wood was found in the wound, and he did need stitches. The elderly nurse who treated him, who, it turned out, was a friend of a late doctor friend of ours, gave him a gentle lecture on using power tools and knowing when to stop driving. I was grateful to her for that.

Close calls are aptly named! Some call them Wake-up calls. Right now I prefer the first name, because I frankly can't live in a state of constant apprehension, if that's what this kind of abrupt, sometimes scary "waking up" calls for.

Yesterday our younger daughter, who works in Manhattan, not far from where eight people were killed by a deranged truck driver on a bike path, said she felt she was becoming desensitized to all the terrorism and violence in the world. I knew what she meant and I wondered, in turn, if I'm becoming desensitized to Ed's close calls.

On the one hand, I hope not. I'm glad I've been near by and can hear Ed and respond to him—thus far—in moments of need.

On the other hand I feel that maybe the underlying message in these four close calls was that, rather than becoming desensitized we must deepen our trust. Our trust in what? In our own intuitions and premonitions. In ourselves and our inner-knowing-what-to-do-when-we-have-to-do it. In our strength to get up and go on when we have to get up and go on, which Ed is doing every day. In our resilience. And in the help that is *always* near—be it in the form of the young man who saw

Ed veer to the left, then to the right in the Jetta, or the TTY and the well-meaning relay operator, or Mr. Manners, or the nurses and doctors in the ER, or who knows whom else we didn't see but who *was* there helping. Like—I do believe—Ed's mother.

Deep Exhaustion ...And Appetite

Close calls—wake up calls—are one thing. Deep exhaustion is another. Deep exhaustion is, to my eye, a far more troubling condition, a condition that can make me feel as powerless as Ed can look.

What exactly do I see when I see it?

I see Ed sitting in his rocker in the living room or on the sofa motionless. Not reading, not listening to the radio, not asking for, or inviting, conversation of any sort. Head a bit bent, eyes on the ground, far off—seeing what?

When it's coming on Ed might say, "I need to sit awhile." Or he'll simply remove himself from what's at hand. Occasionally he lies down on the sofa, or in his chair, feet up on the table. I ask if he needs anything. Water? Tea? Chocolate? His radio? The book he's reading? He'll just shake his head.

It can last 20 minutes, 40 minutes. Then he rouses himself to go back to his desk or out for a walk, as though by walking he can jump-start himself back into daily life. And, as the freezing of gait happens most frequently in our home, he will do his best—sun, rain, mist or snow—to get outside to walk. As though to be sure the sky is still there, or to say hello to the trees and the road, or simply to attempt to breathe O U T- and- A W A Y from it all. There's something about putting one foot in front of the other—left-right, left-right, left-right –that is like a rewinding of some sort that seems to bring the breath back into him, to stabilize him.

When he returns home, 10 or 20 minutes later, he seems reconnected with place, time, body, himself. His eyes meet mine. The smile is back in them.

"Whew!" I think to myself.

Sometimes in the middle of dance class I have seen Al, who has to sit because of this hunched-over back, go out like this. He sits there, looking into space, while we continue dancing beside and around him. As with my Ed, it's as though the air has gone out of him, every bit of invisible, vital, powerful air that holds one up, has suddenly, mysteriously been sucked out of him. You realize a person in this condition *could* fall over and crumple, like a piece of paper, that our breath *does* hold us up.

All the PD books I've leafed through or read through mention fatigue. I didn't pay much attention to that when I first read about it. It made sense to me that dealing with the different symptoms of PD is in itself fatiguing. It takes longer to get everything done, from showering to dressing to eating to typing to getting in and out of the car, to digging one's wallet out of one's back pocket to pay for something. Then there is the work of making oneself understood, dealing with stress or the impatience of others in public places, not to mention right at home! I know when Ed is retreating because he simply hasn't got any "gas" with which to meet the situation. I feel him turning, unconsciously perhaps, to me to provide the gas to keep us both going.

I recently conked out with the 2017-2018 flu. I'm sure many will remember this one. I'd swum my mile at the YMCA when it snuck up on me. I came home, had some lunch, and was working on a pastel when I began to feel cold.

Half an hour later I was on the sofa, beneath a blanket, trying to read the newspaper, and the chills came on full force. More blankets, then the hottest bath I could get into, then into bed with the electric blanket on high. I slept for 12 hours straight and woke in a sweat.

For almost two days, as I alternated between chills and sweats, I had no interest in anything: neighbors, emails, news, books, drink, food (read that as "ice cream"), not even—I will confess—how Ed was going to manage. And he managed fine! It was our dog, Tucker, constantly by the side of the sofa or the bed, within reach of my fingers, who reminded me I'd better not disappear entirely.

When I came out the other end of this flu several pounds lighter, weak, wispy, blinking in the bright light of day, the rumblings in my stomach filled me with wonder. I didn't wake up, put the thermometer in my mouth, read it and then decide, "My temperature's back to normal, so I'm better…." I was hungry, thirsty, awake, eager, inquiring, interested. I <u>was</u> hunger, thirst, wakefulness—all of it! I felt with my whole body how this was, indeed *is*, a pretty amazing thing. A wave— another kind of forceful wave—had carried me back to land. My renewed appetite for life was miraculous.

Yes, I felt keenly how appetite for life is a miraculous thing, a gift. How PD can eat away at it, little by little, day by day, sometimes in great chunks. One minute Ed is walking along the road, doing everything right, apparently eagerly, and his limp right arm is swinging a bit. Ten minutes later he's close to stumbling back to the house and onto the sofa.

We can try and figure it out by the medications schedule—the "peak" times and the "off" times—but such research clearly has its limits. We can try and get some protein into him—a hard-boiled egg, a smoothie, a handful of nuts. If that doesn't work, Coke, coffee or dark chocolate. But more often than not Ed just shakes his head. It's as though the deep exhaustion that is PD is daring him to look *at* it, not to force his way through or dodge his way around it.

This deep exhaustion isn't, I believe, rooted in apathy and hopelessness, though I believe it can lead to both. It is often mistaken for depression. I say mistaken because, even though I know Ed has his depressed moments, I've also seen his pick-up moments. His appetite for life turns back on, sometimes gradually, other times suddenly. A surprise phone call from one of our daughters can get him going again, or a song on the radio, or the bright late afternoon light on the treetops, or a dispute in the yard between bluebird and swallow as to who gets first rights in which bird house.

I think this deep exhaustion is rooted in the physical body. You can call it a chemical aberration or major breakdown. From Ed's point of view it's a nuisance, because all the rest of him wants to keep on keeping on. From the point of view of love, my love for Ed, it's a peep hole into the great mystery of appetite. Even if this deep exhaustion is rooted in the physical body, life also is rooted there. Regardless of what's not working properly, appetite is there calling forth hunger—the hunger that keeps one going.

The Importance of Reconnecting Again
And Yet Again

We had another struggle today with impatience.

Ed said we needed to get the names of some contractors for a repair job, and I said I'd given him one just a few weeks ago. I had, but Ed didn't remember, and the tone in which I replied was all wrong. It probably called up Ed's worry of PD leading to forgetfulness, confusion, possibly dementia.

"I'm put off by the way you're talking," he said.

He was right on.

I did say I was sorry, but fact is I wasn't really sorry. I wanted to get into my day, into other things I was thinking about. I didn't want to be yanked back into another moment of "How PD Has Changed the Way We Live Our Everyday Lives."

I got a copy from the file on my desktop of the email I'd forwarded to Ed with the name of the contractor. Proof that I was right. If he hadn't read it and/or printed it out, well, that was his fault.

I could see from his face that he was still hurt by the way I was talking.

Again I said I was sorry. And I *was* sorry this time. Very sorry.

Ed then commented on how we assume each knows what the other is talking or even thinking about—we've done that for almost 50 years. This knowing has flowed back and forth between us pretty seamlessly. In the last year, though, I've realized it isn't always the case. He asks me what I am talking about, or what I really mean, or am getting at or am trying to get at, and I ask him the same questions. Sometimes I feel I have to go back to step one in order to make clear why we're now at step three. I can lose enthusiasm for whatever we're trying to talk about when we're doing that. I can begin to think, "To heck with contractors." Then that topic, through no fault of its own, becomes charged, something to be avoided. A red flag. Or—if we're lucky—it's turned into a shared joke. Because it *is* possible to turn these misunderstandings, these occasional misconnections, into jokes. It's possible to see the absurdity of allowing the name of a contractor, whom neither of us even know, to ruin our day.

Ed knows he isn't as quick and his thinking isn't as comprehensive as it was in the past. Multitasking—thinking or talking about several different things within the course of a couple of minutes—is plain frustrating. I don't blame him. It's like the way a deaf person attempts to follow and understand crisscrossing conversations. No sooner have you gotten hold of the topic within one group of people than the talk switches to another.

Taking time to think through things, rather than always assuming we're on the same page, is a bit like Ed's difficulty typing. The tremor in Ed's right hand makes it hard for him to hit the right key. The keyboard *can* seem awfully small and tight. The sphere of thinking can, likewise, become smaller and tighter. It all takes more time, more concentration, more control, more energy, more of everything to get it done. The fingers of the mind, to speak metaphorically, have to work harder to make the connections between topics and may hit the wrong keys.

It is said that people with PD can become over-focused, can become obsessed with details, trying the patience of those close to them. An example of this is James in dance class talking on and on about some bit of PD research when we all are beyond wanting to hear about it. We just want the class to begin, but we don't know how to interrupt him without sounding rude or hurtful.

I sympathize when James' wife privately confesses her battle with impatience when James gets going. It happens to me, too. For example, Ed may be tying a couple of boards on top of the car before a 40 minute drive home. Does he *really* need to make double knots? Is it *really* necessary that the little extra bit of dangling rope after he's done has to be tucked way back where no one can see it? Does he think we're driving all the way to Alaska with that wood? I'm shifting my weight from foot to foot, just wanting him to be done so we can get in the car and get going.

To return to the particular moment of impatience I started describing: I had hurt Ed, who in turn hurt me, and likely more than I had hurt him. Because after my second more sincere apology, he seemed to be able to get on with his day, whereas I felt awful. His face when I was impatient—he'd looked momentarily as though I'd hit him.

I couldn't help but remember how I cringed inwardly whenever my father became impatient when having to repeat something or make himself understood to a deaf person (me). He'd slow down and enunciate to the point of unnecessary exaggeration, could make it sound as though I were stupid or mentally deficient.

Do I want Ed to feel that way when I become impatient and repeat things I know I've already told him? Heck, *no!*

Rudolf Steiner's says our thoughts and feelings are as real and powerful as physical actions. We are literally setting energies in motion when we express our thoughts and feelings. And I can see the effect on Ed of the energy behind my words, especially when they're coming not out of caring, respect or consideration, but out of impatience, frustration, even anger.

Every now and then, in a moment of impatience, I have to stop myself.

Am I angry at Ed, really, or am I angry at PD?

Has Ed become the target of anger directed at PD?

What's it like to be angry at PD?

Such anger feels abstract—I can't really *see* PD. I can see its effects, yes: the tremor, festination, stooping, shuffling, slowness, facial mask, loss of energy, loss of confidence. But PD itself, what is that? What is *it*?

Furthermore, is my anger really anger or is it fear?

Is it arising out of a sense of helplessness in the face of the onward march of PD, helplessness that comes and goes, sometimes in a torrent all at once, sometimes in a slow trickle?

One of the most helpful thoughts that came my way recently is that there's something good in fear. Yes, something good. My initial response was, *"Really?"* Sure, fear may be necessary, warning, alerting me to something I need to be aware of. The creepy stranger on the street, the suspicious-sounding email in my inbox, the way the mink in the woods last spring hissed rather than running away.

But isn't fear itself the thing to be feared, the thing that diverts me from or robs of me of my own innermost power? Shouldn't I gird myself daily with faith, hope, gratitude, courage?

The essence of the thought that came my way is that fear is about the future. When I fear this or that will happen, I'm worrying about something I think, feel or imagine might happen in the future, whether that "future" is a day, a month, or months away; something that might not happen. Even, and especially, when what's happening now makes the future look rather bleak, I often tend to imagine the worst. Ed, because he's not home yet, could've been in a car accident or lost his balance and fallen some place. In moments of physical and spiritual exhaustion, I lose my heart's sense of the openness of the future and fill it up with the worst-- way beyond what might actually happen.

Yes, it's important to be in the "here and the now."

Yes, being in the here and now can slow me down and remind me to be grateful for all I have, can open my eyes to the beauty all around me, can cool the wish, ache and greed for more, and yet more.

But the future *is* also important, and even when it feels as though PD has robbed us of the future, I can feel my heart pushing toward it, like a seed in the depths of the dark earth. This future calls out hope and eager expectation. It asks to come into its own—to grow, swell, laugh, dance.

So now there's this other angle to fear to which I never paid much attention. Might fear actually be a cousin of hope? For both call forth expectation and anticipation. Fear can, I'm discovering, be found to call forth longing as well as dread. For there have actually been moments when I've gotten tired of being afraid. Even bored with it. This moment's "bad" really isn't as bad as I'd imagined a month ago. I'm still breathing, Ed's still breathing. We can still look each other in the eyes and smile. But, hey, I want it to be better than this. Less fraught, less wrung out, less paralyzing.

When this happens I feel a movement in me toward courage: the courage to look *at* and *beyond* the fears as they arise, rather than expending a lot of energy trying to suppress them or blot them out. Fear is, after all, mostly about possibilities, usually not so good ones. Yes, I need to be prepared. But rather than giving in to the impulse to paint the possibilities as automatically confining and dark, I need to allow the future to express its essential spaciousness—like an enormous blank canvas on which I can paint anything my heart—not my worried mind—and Ed's heart too, long to paint…

…and see what happens.

When nudged by courage in this way to look *at* the fears and *beyond* them, I have sensed helpful thoughts and feelings coming to me like dear friends and wise visitors.

One is the realization help has *always* come when I have needed it, though not always in the form I might have expected, or at the time I thought I most needed it. Ed and I are not alone.

Another is the knowing that it is important to *ask* when I need help, if not verbally, then from my heart in prayer. And not to worry about bothering others-- whether that other is our next door neighbor, or a friend on the other side, or God!

Yet another is the certainty: this experience of PD that we are having together is but a chapter in our life together—and, damn-it, my intention is for it to be as well-written as possible!

What's most needed in these moments when Ed and I find ourselves out of sync?

It seems to lie in my making a genuine effort to stop and reconnect with my husband—with this great guy named Ed, or Edward, as I sometimes prefer to call him. With myself, too. And with the future, his, mine, ours.

Every now and then, in the middle of what may seem like an ordinary day, there's this need to reconnect.

Last Saturday afternoon and evening, Ed was stumbling about, the festination worse than ever. I asked why it was worse. He admitted that when he was talking on the phone with our younger daughter that morning he'd not taken his 10:30 dose of medication. Had he forgotten, or had he simply not wanted to be bothered to take it? His response made it sound like a combination of both, his version of not wanting to be yanked back into another moment of "How PD Has Changed the Way We Live Our Everyday Lives."

He'd taken the Simenet over an hour late. That meant the Simenet didn't kick in till 30 or 40 minutes later. That in turn threw his mealtimes off, because an hour needs to pass before or after one has taken the Simenet, so he had an energy dip, and when he has an energy dip he's easily discouraged. All this makes for more tension in his back, more stress, more stooped shoulders, more freezing up.

Everything is so much more tightly interwoven than even six months ago. One perfectly understandable moment of wanting to talk with his daughter, without any reminder of PD, led to what looked to me like the possibility of some serious missteps and possibly a fall.

I was briefly angry at him for forgetting to take his medication. He has a vibrating wrist watch to remind him to take the meds every three hours. If that's not enough, am I supposed to be the reminder? How I hate being a nag.

But that flash of anger didn't last more than a moment, because it was clear Ed needed help reconnecting with the schedule that holds him on course. Helping to guide him back into that connection, I also felt better. Less worried. Part of a team, not a nag.

What is this all reconnecting—connecting—reconnecting yet again about, if not Love?

"How Is It with You?"

Often, when we've just left a party, or when one of us steps in the back door when returning from a meeting, a walk or a swim, Ed or I will ask, "How is it with you?" Or, if seeing one another some time later, the query will be in the past tense, "How was it for you?" Other questions lie like nesting dolls within that question: "How *are* you?" "*Where* are you?"(not geographically but in thought or feeling) "Did you miss me?"

I'm sure other couples have their own private and idiosyncratic ways of checking in with one other, and I deeply appreciate how Ed continues to check in with me, even if how things are with him is the paramount question in our lives since now.

For us, as for most couples I'm sure, there has always been this sensitivity to what the other is thinking and feeling. Yes, our thoughts and feelings are often entwined, but one or the other—a thought or a feeling—may dominate. For example, I might pick up on a critical thought Ed is entertaining toward someone, when we're at a meeting or watching the news. It might, if I ask him, translate into, "Whew! What a windbag!" Or Ed's agitation will be evident when he gets up abruptly and leaves the room, but I may have no idea what triggered his sudden exit. This is happening more and more. He's told me he simply can't take in everything in a group conversation and sometimes feels the need to distance himself from everyone. Six or eight people in a room may suddenly be too many.

Ed is not only thinner weight-wise, he is also thinner-skinned. I can relate to that: crying grandchildren sound louder than ever, hot beverages on the lips are hotter than ever, direct sunlight is more blinding than ever. At moments Ed is like the canary in the coal mine. He can only tolerate so much messiness, confusion, and BS. And there are the times when I'm a part of the fumes in his coal mine! He's told me rightly—and more than once—to "cool off" when talking politics, to be a bit less blunt, or to complete my sentences. He was a bit this way prior to the PD diagnosis, but now the little irritations are definitely closer to the surface. We're both retired and may at times agree with the sentiment, "I married you for better or for worse but *not* for lunch every day." Being together so much more than when we were going in different directions to work has ratcheted up our sensitivity to each other's thoughts and feelings.

PD means things have to happen at a slower pace. It takes longer for Ed to do many things: dress, shave, pack, unpack, find the words to clothe his thoughts. He can pick up on my impatience with this, as when I'm sitting in the car in the driveway, ready to go, and he's having a little trouble getting medications, water bottle, satchel, coat, hat, gloves, eyeglasses and cane all in hand to go. Then I can feel his impatience with *my* impatience when he finally gets into the car. And if, at this point, he's hit with a bout of dyskinesia (involuntary bodily movements) who's to blame? It's possible stress is a factor when it comes to dyskinesia. So who is stressing out whom? We can just laugh at the whole thing or — I'll admit this has happened — I drive *very* fast down the hill making Ed nervous, and I'm so relieved we're finally moving, the impatience is left behind, smoldering in the driveway. And, hey — look at the sky today! And Mt. Monadnock way off in the distance has a gorgeous coat of snow! And to heck with PD — we're off to dance class!

I think of this as a double switch. We've both switched into the same emotion (impatience) and switched out of it simultaneously. Now — this is another example of picking up the emotions of a beloved – I think I can hear Ed telling me not to be so confident that he is able to shake off his impatience with me when I shake off mine with him, meaning that his impatience is more justified than mine is. And my response to that? On the one hand, as when driving fast down the hill, I sometimes *like* being prickly or defiant. It's just a need to be contrary every now and then. Ed, too, can be contrary. It's as though, after 50 years together always sleeping on the same sides of the bed, even when not at home, it's time to vary the pattern.

On the other hand, thanks to PD, I'm continually learning that 95 percent of the time we really *don't* have to hurry. Ed doesn't have to catch a train, nor am I about to give birth to a baby. I know that the slower-than-usual pace is *not* something Ed asked for. Over are the days when we gleefully, even vainly, bounded up and over mountains well below the average hiking times given in the guide books. Yes, we were nimble!

There are also times when an overbearing emotion switches, or is transferred, from Ed to me, or from me to him. Ed's discouragement can settle on me. I can feel it on my shoulders, my neck, my back. Discouragement, disappointment and depression are heavy and dark.

They flatten one. Some of these emotions can be very specific. Ed might, for example, tell me about an embarrassing moment he had in Home Depot when he couldn't get cash out of his wallet easily and others were waiting behind him, grim faced and restless. I see it as he describes it, and I feel the mortification of it all. He can begin to sound and look better—indeed lighter—as he's telling me about it, but I feel the weight of it. Hey, wait a second! Do we have to share_everything_?

I know there are times when taking on the feelings of others can be uncalled for, unnecessary and unhealthy. But I don't begrudge Ed giving me these feelings, I _want_ to help lighten his burden. Then there are the times when it's clear that meeting the difficult thoughts and feelings together head-on, admitting their presence and accepting them, can help to transform them. I think of this as turning and facing the wolf that's snapping at your heels when you know you can't outrun it. Now there are two of us, holding hands, facing it down. And very often the "wolf" turns out to be quite a bit smaller and less threatening than I'd imagined. Or maybe it's not a wolf at all; maybe it's just an odd-shaped tree trunk seen from a distance, that only resembles a wild beast.

There are also the times when I sense it's not a matter of lightening Ed's burden, but of protecting us:

You have given me permission
to "have it all out"
though the sharing may not flow easily—
may become a muddy pool
of swirling undercurrents.
As I experienced yesterday
after we went to the doctor,
when his face told me
what I didn't want to hear.

There _are_ times when I know
I must hide my feelings,
hold them in, push them down,
look the other way.
I do not want you to get caught up in them:
fear can be contagious.
Allow me time—

to gauge the whirlpools
on my own.

In a subtle yet humorous way, Ed's frustrations and confusions can be as contagious as fear, as can be seen in an experience I recorded half a year ago in my journal:

Last night I took Ed's car to attend a meeting in Northampton.

I was feeling a little guilty about leaving Ed as he was in the middle of a big computer-frustration meltdown. The medical portal on which he was trying to compose a letter to his doctor kept shutting down before he could complete what he wanted to type. The fact that he kept hitting the wrong keys and had to correct what he'd written ate into the limited time span allowed on the portal. It's clear that composing his letters to the doctor off-line, then pasting them in the portal, would help. But there's no escaping the fact that typing is harder and harder for him, and the word-recognition technology isn't that useful because of the softness of his voice. Perhaps I should offer to type for him. It's ironic that some of these PD doctors who want to help and want to keep their patients up-to-date on new developments aren't aware of some of the difficulties of "new developments"—in this instance medical portals—for folks with PD.

Because I left the house filled with Ed's frustrations with technology, I wasn't fully in what I was doing.

Seated in Ed's VW, eager not to be late for my meeting, I was five miles down the road before I glanced at the gas gauge. And I was thoroughly annoyed: The tank was close to empty! He could've warned me! Should I go back to the house and get my own car or stop at the station near the highway? I decided to stop at the station.

All the pump stations were empty so I had my pick of the lot. I punched in the needed information, put the hose in the car, got one squirt of gas and the hose jerked off abruptly.

I tried again.

Again, the hose jerked off.

Thinking that pump might be broken, I backed up to the pump behind it. Again, I was only able to get a squirt of gas.

92

Puzzled, I ran into the station and told the guy neither pump was working and what should I do? I'd never seen him there before. He looked about 19—a very boyish 19—with a short and bushy crew cut, a plain black tee shirt and an unusually open face.

He said the pump would probably work if I prepaid. I prepaid for $15 dollars worth of gas and went back out.

Again the hose jerked off.

I ran back into the station and asked the guy if he could please help me figure out the pumping. As he was the only worker at the store, he was reluctant to leave it unattended. I pointed out no one was around and I was his sole customer, so he came out to take a look.

The pump would not work for him either, and he directed me to a third pump and offered to fill the car up.

Gas began pouring down the side of the car.

I grabbed the attendant's arm—he was looking at the pump —and he quickly stopped the flow.

We both looked inside the car at the dashboard and burst out laughing! The gas gauge in the VW was at full, *not* at empty! No wonder all the pumps had jerked off.

We were embarrassed but we also couldn't stop laughing. He gave me back $`12 and asked me not to tell his boss about the incident.

As I got back in the car, I realized I'd totally forgotten about Ed and his frustrations communicating by way of the computer. How about me trying to communicate with Ed's VW and the gas pumps?

It also dawned on me as I drove on down to Northampton that I'd been assuming the tank was empty when it really was full. Very full! Was there was a message in that?

No, I haven't lost my marbles. I *can* figure out these little things when I'm attentive to *them*, rather than overly attentive to Ed's moods.

The occasional missteps can be rather funny.

Here's another incident from my journal. This one, however, wasn't funny. This time, when I picked up Ed's anxiety in a public space it felt

93

as though it was happening to me, too.

We went to Northampton to do some Christmas shopping. We both were eager to do as much of it as possible and that, in itself—I realized later—added to the stress. We'd made a list before we went, but though we knew from our girls what the grandkids were hoping to get, Ed wanted to find certain things *by* himself, as gifts *from* himself. I, of course, had my own ideas of what I wanted to get them. In the past we've done much of our Christmas shopping separately.

So there we were in the store, A to Z, which was overflowing with just about every gift you can think of for children of all ages; overflowing also with other grandparents and parents in gift-hunting mode.

Because of the crowd, I kept circling back to Ed to see how he was doing and suddenly there he was standing in a small aisle, heavily stocked shelves on either side, and I could see he had frozen up. There was a look of utter uncertainty on his face. Where to go? How to get going?

In that minute, I froze, too (he didn't know I was looking at him). It was claustrophobic! The shoppers pressing all around, the shelves up to the ceiling, the close air, the absence of natural light, the narrow aisle. In that minute I felt, physically, how Ed must feel when the festination hits. Immobilized, trapped, spaces closing in… and in… and in.

All I knew was that we had to get out of there! I rushed forward to help him before he stumbled.

"BIG step!" I whispered as I took his hand.

It was as though his right leg heard me and moved right into step with my right leg.

Outside, walking back to the car, we both breathed a big sigh of relief. So what if we were empty handed. So what if we had to plan another trip there at a less-crowded time. Moments like this bring home what's *really* important. Being able to move freely, all the money in the world can't buy that back. Being able to move freely *within* oneself; calmly, without anxiety, with trust that the way can be found.

Later I realized I've gone beyond caring how people look at

us. Why do we need to try to "normalize" everything, especially when things aren't normal, aren't right? There was something liberating in that realization.

Now, one last story from my journal, also not a funny account. It took us both a couple of steps closer to one of the scarier possibilities for those with PD: cognitive decline.

Ed and I were having dessert when the phone rang. It was Kristina, our hair cutter, calling to reschedule my appointment for the next day. After Ed had conveyed her message and Kristina and I had agreed on another time, I went out to the kitchen with the dinner dishes. And so the evening chores flowed into one another.

When I went upstairs to my desk Ed came up to say the phone was missing and where had I put it? It was the cordless phone he'd used when speaking with Kristina. (I don't use it because I can't hear on the phone.)

I went downstairs with Ed and we looked for it, unsuccessfully, on the first floor and in the basement. I returned to my desk upstairs to continue what I'd been working on.

Next thing, Ed was going around the house unplugging the other phones in order to hear the ring of the missing one when he called the house via his cell phone. A good idea but, despite two or three tries, he didn't hear anything, nor did I.

When I went to say good night Ed asked, "Where did *you* put the phone?"

It's been a joke of ours when he asks, with a grin in his eyes and a wag of his finger, where I've hidden something when he can't find it. This joke began years ago when he once left his eyeglasses on the dining room table and I put them in the bouquet of flowers in the middle of the table, hidden, yet in easy sight if you looked carefully. But the missing phone wasn't a joking matter. It was symbolic of the things he's been forgetting or losing in private and public places: keys, gloves, cane, wallet, cell phone, sweat shirts and yes, eyeglasses.

He was genuinely rattled. That, in turn, rattled me. We know that plenty of older folks without PD experience memory loss and gaps of one sort or another—I certainly do—but there was an edge, a sharpness, to Ed's response I hadn't felt before. This sharpness felt, momentarily, like a form of despair amounting to: "DAMN!! I've already given up so much to PD—must I lose my mind too?" And I felt unable to offer any real reassurance.

Later, shortly after I'd gone to bed, Ed came up to our bedroom to tell me he'd found the phone in the cupboard beneath the TV. He looked immensely relieved, even triumphant. He'd figured out he'd put it there, along with the remote control for the TV, after Kristina had called.

By then, however, I was unable to drift off to sleep. The realization had slipped in that there may come a time when we can't just talk things over, reconnect, put our chins up again and paddle on till the next big wave hits. There might come a time when we're no longer in the same boat.

Every now and then Ed has difficulty expressing himself. Two medical terms for this, one of which I mentioned earlier, are:

Dysphonia: difficulty producing a strong or clear voice.

Dystonia: abnormal, involuntary movement that results from the simultaneous contraction of muscle(s) that have opposing actions. Dystonic movements are slow, cramped, and usually follow a repeating pattern. (from Navigating Life with PD, information on this book is on page 153)

Ed's way of describing this difficulty when it's happening and I ask is that he can't fit thoughts to words and words into sentences. This sounds— I described it a bit in the earlier chapter on Funny Mouth Movements--and looks like a muscular mix-up with his tongue sometimes getting in the way of his lips, which makes it harder for me to speech-read him. I have to ask him to repeat or rephrase what he's trying to say, and that, in turn, can cause more stress and freezing up.

After years of Ed having to interpret for me—the deaf one—I'm now sometimes being put in the position of having to interpret for him. Fifty years of being able to pick up easily, often without any words, what the other is thinking and feeling is being challenged in subtle ways. I am humbled by how hard it can be, how a direct and automatic "What did you say?" may not be the best way to go. Can he give me the topic rather than repeating the sentence word for word? Can he point at something or act out his thought? Are there new ways I can attune to him to understand where he is and how it is for him? There must be! And I do think our dance class is key here. The mirroring, the improvising, the humor and the music all help to lighten and loosen us up. Could it also be that, PD or no PD, the ways we communicate with the people we are closest to change with time? Why wouldn't they change? I'm learning, through "How is it for you?", one cannot assume anything when it comes to communicating, even and especially with my own husband.

Concerns around cognitive clarity are also heightened when I see the drug literature Ed brings home from the pharmacy with his prescription refills: warnings of forgetfulness, sleepiness, dizziness and more. I glance over these papers, forget what I've read, reread them, toss them out. We find the warnings scary. The same cautious notifications are in the books. We don't want to spend our days worrying and wondering about what might happen when taking this or that drug, and if this or that drug is behind an "off" time, yet we *do* want to be fully alert to what's going on.

Here's where our connection with Ed's PD doctor is so important. Dr. S is two and a half hours away, and he wants Ed to check in with him every four months, so our visits to him are usually all day excursions. (Talking with him on the phone and emailing with him are nowhere near as satisfying.) Sometime there's a longer-than-usual wait to see him, but that's okay with us because he's completely *with* us when we're with him. He is on the young side, and his listening is keen, thoughtful, light, light in the sense of not being overburdened by having to listen day in and day out to folks with PD.

We're grateful not only for the generous amount of time and information he shares with us but also and especially for the reach of his awareness. He isn't just thinking about the brain and the missing dopamine; he's thinking about diet, the stomach, weight, exercise, physical fitness, personality, individual initiative, family care and more. And thank God, he has a sense of humor. He even wondered aloud one time about possibly starting a clinical trial for people with PD that would involve fly fishing! We see Dr. S as an ally rather than an all-knowing expert, and almost always come out of our meetings encouraged and energized.

"How was that for you?" Ed asks after we've lined up the next appointment at the check-out station.

"Good. For you, too?"

Ed usually nods.

Later we'll go over the details of Dr. S's responses to our observations and questions, and our responses to his suggestions or recommendations. We often discover we had the *exact* same inner response at the *exact* same moment during an appointment.

This happened recently, after Ed had described some bothersome new PD symptoms. Dr. S paused for a moment, looked at Ed, looked at me, then looked again at Ed and very gently said, "Well...it sounds as if the honeymoon is over."

"*What* honeymoon?" was my inner response, and Ed's too, I learned later, as we were walking back to our car.

"I married you, I *didn't* marry PD!" Ed declared.

"Same here," I agreed, "You and I are the married ones. What's a PD honeymoon anyway?"

Of course, we both knew Dr. S meant Ed had entered a more advanced stage of PD. In our minds and hearts, we already knew this and we had perhaps been dreading that Dr. S would confirm it. But the way he chose to do so had, for me, at least, taken the edge off the shock of having it articulated out loud. It was actually a good distraction from a chunk of discouraging news. Honeymoon? Really? Come on! How could *any* part of the PD experience be called a honeymoon? (Later we gathered that other PD doctors use that expression to explain to their patients that the very helpful effects of Sinemet when one first goes on it are, unfortunately, wearing off.)

Above all, Dr. S conveys a sense of onwardness, the sense that life continues even as it comes at us with scary new symptoms; and he also conveys the importance of our meeting PD to the best of our ability with the best tools he can recommend or make available. I believe this *onwardness* is rooted in the virtue of keeping on keeping on.

Dr. S's appreciation of Ed moves me deeply. I know he sees Ed, the Ed I see. His interest in Ed comes across as a form of hope, hope that science will gradually find and fit together the many different parts of this foreboding, jagged puzzle that's PD.

"How is it with you?"

There are times when I can only ask Ed that question in my thoughts or through my eyes, because I see he's down, disappointed, feeling out of the flow of life, weary of having to give so much energy physically to keeping going physically. There are moments when we're frankly sick and tired of talking about PD. A cheery and well-meaning, "How _are_you?" from a neighbor can actually feel intrusive, as if that person is asking for a detailed report on the last month and a half since our paths last crossed. "How are you _today_?" is easier to handle. And distractions are welcomed, even political distractions! It can feel good to be angry at something else, some outrageous mess, someone out there who truly rubs you all wrong.

When we first got the diagnosis, and for a couple of years afterward, I felt a need, almost a responsibility, to help Ed stay "up", as though being "down" was a failure on his part or mine. I hated the awkward silence that would descend when friends or family got a glimpse of the festination or when Ed quite clearly didn't know what to say, and because of that, pulled back, and because of the PD mask didn't look very approachable. People who didn't know what was going on turned to me, evidently puzzled. And how was that for me? A little scary. I didn't want to be Ed's mouthpiece. And I still don't want to be his mouthpiece, but now it's for a different reason. It feels so important that _his_ voice continue to be heard, that _he_ share how it is with him as often as possible. Deafness taught me the importance of being heard—and seen—first hand. Advocating for oneself is, I believe, an important part of one's identity.

Now, 10 years after the diagnosis, it's clear the "down" times are, like the seasons of the year and the phases of each day, a part of this journey. They are to be weathered, waves to roll with rather than to flee. And Ed _has_ endured them, _is_ enduring them. I am learning first hand, by being with him, what true strength is.

Almost every morning Ed and I sit together for a few minutes, light a candle, read something inspiring and send blessings to others, or pray for the well being of our country, our earth, whomever or whatever comes to mind. This time feels as important as breakfast, it is, indeed, a kind of breakfast. It can seem as though family and dear friends, both here and on the other side, are with us, sitting or standing beside us, sharing smiles, occasionally winking, observing with us a moment of quiet and deep thanks before we step into a new day.

When we're specifically concerned about someone—like a sick grandchild—it sure makes *me* feel better (meaning less worried) to say a prayer for that child. And when we're concerned about a specific situation, like, for example, the victims of yet another shooting, a profound certainty settles on me: *Every true prayer from the heart matters, is heard, is taken, is a balm and medicine, makes a difference.* And I know that others are sending prayers Ed's way, our way, and it's important that we not only acknowledge, take, give thanks, but also send out love, so it can go on, and on.

Give and it shall be given unto you, good measure, pressed down, and shaken together, and running over.

Of Woods and Wood

We went to our favorite swimming spot yesterday only to find it was closed, because a thunderstorm had left the river unusually high and stirred up. So, instead, we walked around the grassy picnic area, and while skirting the puddles we noticed a path snaking into thick undergrowth. Where did it go? The old hiker's urge to follow it hit both of us, and into the forest we went in our bathing suits and sneakers, without a moment's hesitation.

The trail led alongside a stream, then up the side of a small hill. Then it went further into the woods, away from the stream, then up and up another eroding hill. The rain-soaked ground was sandy in some spots; in others it was slippery with fallen, glistening leaves. Bright chartreuse clumps of grass and jewelweed had taken hold and sprouted fountain-like where sunlight seeped through. Ed seemed uncertain of his footing at several points and grabbed at stumps, tree branches and sapling trunks. The height and uneven footing made him unsure of his balance. I regretted that he didn't have one of his canes to steady him and looked around unsuccessfully for a walking stick. But on he went, determined to reach the top.

Though the area was somewhat disheveled—no other folks were in sight— there was nothing dark or sinister about these woods. Young beeches, aspens, cottonwoods, junior and senior maples, but not many evergreens. Layer upon layer of green leaves rustled overhead and floated around us like hearts, opened hands, paws, feathers, all freshly washed, healthy, thriving, welcoming.

In the 10 or 15 minutes it took us to scramble up that hill, I was taken back through half a dozen rainy-day rambles in the White Mountains of New Hampshire, a walk in the Olympic National Forest in Washington, a hike among the shiny red-skinned Pacific Madrone of the San Juan islands, and other wet walks in Connecticut, upstate New York, Scotland and the Audubon sanctuary beside our home.

Ed was leading, as he always did when we hiked, setting the pace, exclaiming over unusual trunk shapes, the tenacity of roots, the persistence of younger trees, the quiet strength of older ones. ("Think of the energy

101

of that oak there, holding its arms up and out day after day.")

Our spur-of-the-moment hike through these lovely, unfamiliar — yet oh so familiar — woods was like a sudden sprint out ahead of the daily grind of PD. Despite the need now and then to steady himself, it struck me from behind him that Ed's total absorption in where he was next going to put his foot, how he was going to get "up there," made for movements that looked completely "normal." It was as though the woods had taken us both back in time: me to my memories and Ed into his White Mountains body. Briefly I felt exhilarated by the thought that regular hikes could help counter his festination. Briefly I imagined us doing sections of the Appalachian Trail or even going back to Scotland!

At the top of the steep hill, clear blue sky opened up overhead. We waded through more jewelweed and patches of giant goldenrod and giant milkweed onto a dirt road. Directly ahead of us was a fenced-in, crew-cut baseball field. In the distance beyond it was yet another green fenced-in field. We were evidently in the dumping area behind the playing fields. There were mounds of bulldozed earth covered with crabgrass, enormous uprooted tree trunks and felled, dismembered trees.

The scene was for me a let-down after the beauty of the woods: no view out over the river where we swim, or Mt. Washington or Mt. Rainer in the distance. But Ed, though weary and drenched with sweat, was still in an exploratory frame of mind. He wanted to see if there was another, easier path back down to the swimming area (there wasn't). He also wanted — actually *needed* — to take a look at the felled trees.

For as long as I've known him, Ed has been not just a lover of trees but an equally ardent lover of wood, and a woodworker as well. Though an educator by profession (teacher, assistant head, headmaster, founder and director of two schools), he could easily have been an architect or a designer and maker of furniture. He did, in fact, take one semester off from teaching when in his thirties to take orders for various pieces of furniture he made in our small basement: coffee tables, beds, bookshelves, small bureaus, music stands, a candelabrum, regular chairs and a hefty rocking chair with a secret compartment behind the seat in which to hide valuables. However, finding the right wood, or being surprised by the changing nature of the wood, or having difficulties with machinery or even difficulties with customers, proved too challenging and he returned to teaching. But woodworking became a hobby that's still very much alive.

Now, instead of furniture, he's often making toys for our grandkids. One Christmas he made a wooden car for each member of the family and each car had hooks at either end so all the cars could be linked up as one train. He designed and built a sturdy playhouse that had the grandkids, and the cousins of the grandkids, wanting to saw and hammer alongside him. His special interest now, though, is the lathe, and he's constantly on the lookout for wood with an unusual grain, especially soft, green wood, to turn into bowls or plates.

So here was Ed, eagerly examining a jumble of felled logs. To my eyes that jumble was a rather sad sight: the trees could be forgotten friends and neighbors dumped out of sight, left to rot however they landed. But Ed wasn't seeing them that way at all. I wondered if we were going to be bringing our car here later to haul something away for him to experiment with on the lathe. Ed pointed out some red pine, and now that he'd pointed it out, I *could* see its beauty, its rich, warm coloring. But it looked as though it weighed a ton, and we already have quite a bit of "rescued" wood in the garage and the basement.

As though hearing my thoughts, Ed said the wood wasn't the right sort for the lathe, and after examining a few other tree trunks, we started walking back to the swimming area by way of the road. The PD gait returned as we went along, Ed stumbling a bit and freezing up once or twice. Wishing again that he had a cane, I looked for and then found an adequate walking stick. Another bit of wood and the woods to help him along.

When we were back in the parking lot, it was clear he was weary as he leaned back in the passenger seat and took a deep drink from the water bottle. But both of us were filled up with our little adventure, sweet with the flavor of past expeditions and bushwhacking jaunts off the beaten path.

Later, home again, I asked Ed what it is he so loves about wood and woodworking. I had never thought to ask, because his love is so obvious, not only as he works but in the results.

"You're giving something a second life," was his immediate response.

"You *always* get something back from wood," he continued, "It serves, it's responsive, it's perhaps the most useful natural material to man—and the less you tamper with it, the more it gives, the more it reveals. And," he continued on a roll now, "the grain can be *so* alive! You feel its strength, it's resilience as you're working with it. Even a fallen tree, a tree that seems to be of no apparent use, can fertilize the earth. You're always learning from it."

Family Times

It's about 3:00 am, my usual wake-up-and-worry time. It's as though Worry sees me lying there in bed, free from distractions, not about to go anywhere, and gleefully exclaims, "Ah! Great! I'll pay her a visit right now!"

Ed's asleep, it's mid-August, it's hot (damn hot, in fact) and I'm thirsty. As I reach for the glass of water on the bedside table I remember we aren't at home. We're at my father's summer house upstate New York, with our girls, their husbands and our grandchildren. Remembering they're with us gives me the needed oomph to slam the door on Worry!

"Out, Worry! I'm not going to stew over the meds now! I've given enough time to your chatter about the scary aside effects of that new drug. Ed's balance may be a bit off but I see that and he knows it. PD is *not* going to knock him off the dock into the lake."

Worry slinks away, and hilarious memories from the day before flow in like a cool breeze.

We were mostly in the lake cooling off. There was a moment when Ed and I were sitting on the dock, Laurel and Christa, our daughters, standing in the water near us in their bright bathing suits (Christa in orange, Laurel in pink and black) chatting with us, as their youngest children jumped from the dock into their mother's arms. Lulu and Wynn, both four, jumped in, scurried up the ladder and then jumped again, and yet again. Ah, the joy of those repetitive actions: jumping, splashing, kicking, yelling, being caught by strong mother arms!

I can see Wynn on the dock now, preparing to jump, yet hesitating, looking very wet and skinny, like a half-drowned pup.

Lulu, in the lake in her mother's arms, started chanting, "Jump Wynn! Jump Wynn! *Jump Wynn!*"

A minute later Wynn jumped, just as Lulu was chambering back up the ladder to urge him on.

Now Wynn was in the water in his mother's arms and Lulu began shouting, "Wynn catch me! Wynn catch me! *Wynn catch me!*"

Wynn stared at her. The expression on his face was priceless! It said, *"What am I supposed to do?"*

We both, and Laurel and Christa, laughed until there were tears in our eyes. Is this how it went in the Garden of Eden? One very determined woman and a guy who never quite knew what she was up to?

I remembered earlier yesterday, when Ed was working on the playhouse he designed and had been building bit by bit all summer out by the apple and plum trees. All the grandchildren wanted to help and their cousins who dropped by to play also had to be involved, so Ed set up a makeshift table with bits of scrap wood for them to saw and hammer nails into. Seven or eight kids were busily scribbling crayon marks on wood, sawing, hammering and yelling, "I need a hammer! My turn with the hammer!" Then suddenly, "*Where* are the nails?"

Yup, where were the nails?

As I was looking for the nails in the grass, I spotted deer poop, and two of the kids were barefoot. Were the kids going to get some awful disease? And what about deer ticks? I hadn't given any thought to that.

Laurel and Christa came out to see what the yelling was about and when I pointed out the deer poop they just laughed. Obviously these full-time working mothers have more serious issues to contend with: seamless child care at home when they have to travel for their jobs, husbands who need a break from holding the fort, half a dozen different schedules to juggle, news of bullying and school shootings, foul language in the air…

"Deer poop looks very much like something chocolate," Laurel observed.

"Milk chocolate or dark chocolate?" Christa chimed in.

We were laughing again.

We agreed the poop should be cleaned up yet found only two or three nails while doing that.

"Where are the nails?" an impatient cousin yelled.

"Hey," said Christa, "I think I know…"

She reached out, grabbed Wynn, patted down his shorts and, sure enough, he'd emptied the contents of the nail jar into his pocket. There were pebbles and pennies mixed in with the nails. (He collects *everything!*)

Just then Freya, Wynn's seven-year-old sister, came out bearing snacks on a tray: goldfish crackers, grapes, paper cups and lemonade. Her timing was perfect! Earlier she'd been hunting throughout the yard for wild flowers and then arranging them in tiny bouquets to put around the house. Last weekend when her great uncle took all the grandchildren out for breakfast and Wynn spilt his chocolate milk Freya not only helped clean it up, she offered to share hers with her brother. Here is one who not only asks how she can help but *sees* where help is needed.

Yet another moment from the day appeared before I drifted back to sleep:

Ellie, our eldest grandchild at eleven, slipping onto the picnic bench beside me at supper, close enough to be asking for a hug. I put an arm around her. She's very huggable. I marvel at how much and how widely she reads, but of course her mother and aunt were avid readers and still are. (My yearly Christmas wish to them and their husbands is: Give me a book you discovered this past year.) I marvel too at the range of topics Ellie and I discuss: civil rights, gay and transgender rights, dating, technology, movies, karma and reincarnation. I don't remember talking with my grandparents, or with my parents, about any of those things. In my family, back then, it was said children were to be seen, not heard.

What's really central though, in my conversations with Ellie (and our other grandchildren too, though the youngest don't always remember) is how she looks at me full face when she speaks, as her mother has taught her to do from a very young age. Both Laurel and Christa have always met me where I am, as a deaf person. As children they would even put hearing aid batteries in their ears and walk around, heads bent sideways, pretending to be deaf. Because of their very matter-of-fact acceptance of my hearting loss I know I am safe with them, and sometimes when they catch me bluffing, I feel almost too transparent! Now as PD sucks us backward into roiling waves and tight, dark, worried spaces, our daughters, their ever-helpful husbands and their children continually draw us outward, onward into the world of today, into laughter, into life.

Sometimes at 3:00 am I've thought how nice it would be to live closer to one or the other daughter or—better yet—both. We don't live closer to them because we love where we live and have found our way into a great network of PD resources. Laurel, our first-born, is eight hours away by car, Christa three hours away, but they are just a good thought or an email away, anytime of day or night. I don't like to burden them with our PD concerns, but it is usually to them that I turn when there's been a close call or a new wave of symptoms.

As to how they see us: Recently, when we were together, we sat down and I asked them a few questions about their experience of our PD journey. For even though we only see them four or five times a year, they are on this journey with us and have observations, insights and thoughts that may be of interest to other families in our position. Here follow some notes and quotes I collected.

I began our conversation expressing curiosity about what they remembered of the time they learned their father had been diagnosed with PD.

"I'll never forget it!" was Laurel's immediate response. "We were visiting you in Shelburne from Brooklyn to celebrate your wedding anniversary. Ellie was eleven months old, and we'd hired someone to babysit while Bernie and I joined you and others at the celebration at a nearby restaurant. I remember you two taking Bernie and me aside and sharing the news. I was very concerned, as I could see how nervous and sad you were. I hadn't yet observed any major symptoms, but I could see this was something you were processing, each in your own way. I also remember in the early years, Daddy wondering what people thought was the matter with him, especially if he was tired or showing symptoms in a context where people were not aware of the diagnosis. I *never* want him to be ashamed of having the disease! He deserves support and sympathy and above all, respect for who he is. Easy for me to say, I realize, but still…"

"I was at work when Pops called about transportation plans for the anniversary party, and he mentioned the diagnosis to me," Christa picked up the story. I went into a conference room to talk privately and afterwards went home early, needing time to process. Thor and I had sensed something was off with Pops, so it wasn't a complete shock, but at that moment I knew this diagnosis was going to change our life as a family substantially, and obviously Pops's life *very* substantially."

Christa remembered it was hard getting ahold of what the diagnosis really meant. I believe what she was trying to say was, "How do I fit what's happening to my father in with what I've heard about PD?" For, when talk about a disease comes up in the news we often pick up the "tone" that accompanies it, and the tone when PD is in the news often tends to be rather grim.

She added, "I remember feeling at first that I should mourn but then realizing this PD process could be long. I felt we were lucky in some ways to have the time, as is not often the case with other serious illnesses. So, instead, it was about adjusting. In addition, in the first few years after the diagnosis I felt as though Pops had decided to be clear with those around him of his love for them: his openness and candor felt like an unexpected gift."

Ed and I were both touched by this remark. When Ed heard it he was close to being teary.

I asked Laurel and Christa if they get a strong sense of the progression of PD every time they see their father. Christa's reply matched Ed's and my experience. "It seems like a disease that can cause rapid changes over several months, but mostly there are long periods when not that much is different. I think of those as the plateaus, where Pops has figured out the combination of exercise and medication to hold that as a normal. Then something new emerges, and there's a learning curve, or an adjustment period, until that's the new normal."

She said something we had often wondered about ourselves but had never articulated. "To be honest, I don't have a clear sense of where we are in the progression. Yes, *where is Pops **now** in the progression of PD?* With H [Christa's step- father-in-law who died from Lewy body dementia] the decline was so fast it was obvious he was losing functionality rapidly, and completely. With Pops it feels as though there are many ups and downs around the changes."

Later we learned there are several rating scales that attempt to describe the progression of PD. One scale developed in the 1960's suggests that are five stages to the disease based on worsening motor symptoms. The symptoms given range from a tremor on one side of the body, to increased stiffness and rigidity, to difficulty with balance, to being unable to get up from a bed or chair. This scale seems inadequate to us. If a doctor applied it to Ed now we think he would say Ed is somewhere in the middle.

"Well... " Christa said, "I have real admiration for how you're always looking to improve, rather than settling into resignation."

Laurel and I both nodded in agreement.

"It's as though the PD comes in fits and starts," said Laurel. "Sometimes the progression is clear and the changes are obvious, sometimes less so. Sometimes you both warn me and I don't find it as obvious as you might think. Other times I observe changes myself and am struck by them. I wonder a lot about what will happen in the coming years. I think you two have done an amazing job managing the disease to date, but I also have the sense that this is where it gets more complicated. What treatments will you pursue? What will be compromised most? What trade-offs will there be and how will you make them? "

I agreed that this is where it gets more complicated. The symptoms have worsened, the festination is more frequent and intense and the exhaustion more prevalent.

"Can you hear the changes on the phone when you talk with your father?" I asked.

"Sometimes I can," said Laurel. "But often it seems as if we're having a normal conversation. I'm sensitive to how Daddy feels about PD, so I don't want to dwell on the difficulties when talking on the phone and make him feel self-conscious. As with any of us, the conversations can be shorter or longer, more focused or more distracted, depending on his state of mind and level of fatigue."

 Christa agreed. She paused and then said, "I'm aware when talking on the phone of the emotional side of all this. I can hear the frustration behind Pops's words when he says managing the PD takes so much time and energy, and how that's narrowed his world. In addition, in the last few years I've noticed how he doesn't reach out as much as he once did, which I don't take personally. I take it as an indicator of low energy and how isolating a chronic disease can be."

Both girls said they are very aware of PD in others—any place, any time, in public—and they want to learn more about it.

"I can spot it right away,"said Christa. "I can see it in the way a person moves or how a person holds his body, or the blankness of a face. I'm interested in staying up-to-date on what the evolving treatment options are. I know that depression can be a real side effect of the disease, but most of the discussion is on figuring out how to optimize the medicine. Pops's emotional life must need support too."

 "I'm definitely more aware of PD than I was before the diagnosis, "Laurel said. "Many friends have parents or in-laws with PD, and I often find myself in conversation with them about the disease and how it's affecting our loved ones."

Laurel mentioned that she was much helped by reading, *Brain Storms: The Race to Unlock the Mysteries of Parkinson's Disease*, by Jon Palfreman, as it gave her a good picture of the disease. She tracks what we share about doctor visits, and what's happening at a given moment, but she is interested too in what the emerging treatments are, and the latest thinking about how PD manifests and progresses. "It's such a mysterious disease," Laurel added. "It doesn't seem to affect any two people in exactly the same way."

Both girls said they sometimes worry about Ed's frame of mind.

"Staying positive, not getting discouraged is hard —but clearly *so* critical," Laurel summed it up.

Christa added, "I appreciate and admire how you both talk things through. I have a real sense of the honesty between you two, but I also think the intensity of the day to day must be exhausting. Mumma, the story of your trip to Florida and Pops losing his wallet made me aware of how consuming PD is, and how things fall on you that never have before. I often wish you got more help—what that looks like I don't know. It may be as simple as being willing to ensure that you have a driver at certain times, or support in airports. It's very important that you be clear with Laurel and me how we might help as well."

When I asked if they had advice for people with a family member or close friend recently diagnosed with PD both girls were quick and clear in their responses.

"I'd say, connect with resources like *Brain Storms*," Laurel advised, "and other accessible descriptions of PD, including how it manifests and what is known and what is not. Beyond knowledge of PD, I'd say the biggest thing I would recommend is having patience and knowing there will be lots of twists and turns to the disease. I can see how having a good network of support is essential. That includes everything from the day-to-day support such as Mumma provides to the larger circle of friends, family, PD groups, doctors and therapists who encourage and guide the patient on his journey."

"Setting up space to talk as a family is important," Christa put in." I've so appreciated what I feel is an open, ongoing dialogue between you two, and both of us and Bernie and Thor too about what is happening. For a new diagnosis I would recommend people think about this as the beginning of a long run. You need endurance as it isn't just the first shock of learning about a life-changing condition, it is a slow shift of reality. What's hard is that it isn't clear how long the race is, so pacing and self-care for all are important. I also think it is hugely important to have fun things to focus on: I value the adventures we've all had together, like going to Vieques for Christmas, family time at the summer house, trips to the circus. Let's be sure to continue to share new, fun experiences together. They're so important. They keep us in the present moment."

Then, Christa went in another direction, "PD shows me how the process of aging isn't easy, and our bodies can betray us at some point. It has highlighted for me how lucky I am to be able-bodied and healthy, while I know that isn't forever. And something else, I've wondered is whether Pops pushed himself so hard in his work life he became more vulnerable to PD. Having inherited this tendency to put my all into work, I'm now thinking more deeply about what it means to have more balance in everyday life, especially for the sake of my own family."

Laurel added a few last words. "Our experience with PD has made me more committed than ever to being present in the here and now. There is so much to worry about these days, not only with PD but in the broader world, and there is so little we can control. Making sure we have time to be together, and being fully present when we are, are essential. These times together are very special to me."

They are certainly very special for us too! We always look forward to being with our daughters and their beloveds and feel extremely lucky to have a family like ours. We wish the same for every person we meet with PD.

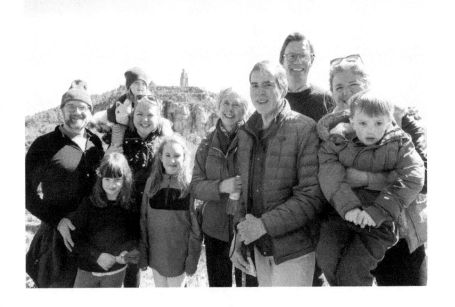

Blatchford Family Photo.
Here we are on our 50th wedding anniversary
ten years after the PD diagnosis.

Looking Back
on Ten Years of Living with PD

Ed is a different person for having lived for over ten years with PD. Older, wiser, thinner, braver, more and more kind. Also, more open and honest with those he loves, both more eager and more wistful, and more prone to help himself to my favorite ginger ice cream after I've gone to bed!

I'm a different person too. Hopefully a more patient, less-in-a-hurry person. I used to think I wanted to be a singer in my next life. After one life time being profoundly deaf, I would get to immerse myself in music. Despite my hearing loss, I love music—the inner music I sometimes hear and the outer music I sometimes hear as well. But I don't know how to read, recognize and appreciate music as it deserves to be appreciated. The human voice in particular has always moved me deeply. I've often wished I could sing from the center of my being with amazement, joy and gratitude.

But now I think I'll fill out a different application for my next life: an application to be a doctor caring for patients or doing research. I'm not sure yet which box I'll check—maybe both! Aren't the two in a way the same? Isn't a doctor's care also a form of research? And isn't the purpose of that research to discover ways to deliver more care-filled, focused care? For me, there's a wish not only to help alleviate suffering— physical, psychological and spiritual—but to understand the connections between the many parts of ourselves—body, soul and spirit—and their connections, in turn, with the warp and woof of the world. I believe this is what today is called integrative medicine.

It has come home to me again and again these past ten years, while learning to roll with the waves of PD, how important it is to be curious. Yes, curious about the PD condition: What does this symptom mean? What's the best diet for Ed, especially when he needs quick energy? Are there ways in our every day life we can map out and explore the concept of neuroplasticity?

Speaking of neuroplasticity, PD is basically about the absence of dopamine in the physical brain and the disorders that result from that.

Readers may wonder why I have not spoken of the surgical treatment for PD called deep brain stimulation (DBS). DBS was approved by the FDA in 2002 and has been beneficial to many, but it is by no means the answer for everyone with PD. At this point, having discussed it with our doctor, we think the downsides of DBS for Ed could outweigh the possible advantages. A major downside could be increased difficulty speaking, as the device is implanted very close to the speech center in the brain. In addition, DBS does not stop the progression of PD. (You can read about DBS in several of the PD books listed at the end of this book.)

When I look into Ed's eyes every morning, and one or the other of us says that wonderful line from John Donne, "And now good morrow to my waking soul" we both know each of us is *much* more than a physical brain with or without a tank full of dopamine. That knowledge, in turn, calls forth more questions in me: Do we human beings have a mind—a center of consciousness—within ourselves apart from our physical brain? Where might this center of consciousness reside, and how might one connect with it? And doesn't this center of consciousness continue even after the physical body has been laid aside? Ed sometimes rolls his eyes when I get going with questions of this sort, but they are questions that not only intrigue me but also make my heart hopeful.

This asking of questions has kept Ed and me active, has led us to insights, resolutions, and the feeling of doing rather than drowning. In the same way that Ed's first PD doctor said, "Use it or lose it" when urging him to keep active physically, we've worked to remain inquisitive in response to this turbulent ocean we've landed in. In my introduction I mentioned that, when exploring pastels, I discovered how the dark colors anchor and make the light colors more real and vivid. Similarly, these past ten years, PD has anchored my awareness and appreciation of life-giving forces everywhere, around and within us.

These forces—and my hope is that this book comes across as a testament to our discoveries —cannot "cure" Ed of PD, but they offer ongoing healing. Curing means restoring to health and normalcy, and—as far as I know—there is no cure for PD. But healing *is* possible, as long as one can stand straight in one's sovereignty, making an effort to see where one is, choosing how one responds and never being afraid to ask for help. Healing, in our experience, doesn't mean returning to a former state. It means knowing ourselves to be connected with the whole of life as it moves onward, no matter the condition one finds oneself in.

In case you wonder, not all the questions we ask are open, earnest or hopeful. There are times when flavor and color seem to evaporate, times when the PD is relentless, ugly, stifling, and Ed may think, "Why did this happen to me?" I asked that too as a deaf kid when having a miserable time in school, and not just once. Yet, somewhere along the way, the question metamorphosed itself into "What can I learn from deafness?" And that question, in turn, has over many years transformed itself into the realization, "I have found help and help has found me. How can I, in turn, be of help to life?"

I see the same thing happening to Ed as he rolls with each wave, often meeting the wave headlong, other times being pulled under for awhile, then reemerging, and always, *always*, when he reemerges, expressing gratitude. When I see, and hear, this gratitude two other things come home to me. The first is how many of the feelings that accompany the daily news are similar to the feelings that come with PD. Feelings of contraction, shrinking, retreat, confusion, frustration, anger, helplessness. In a curious way PD has become, for me, a metaphor of what is going on all around in these unsettled and unsettling times.

The second thing that comes home to me is that *everything* we need to stay afloat every time another enormous wave comes along *can* be found if we can remain thankful. As I know from living with him, Ed's gratitude is the light that rises up from beneath each dark wave.

My Story, So Far

I thank Claire for writing these sketches of our journey with Parkinson's over the past decade. She asked me to add a final section from my perspective as the one who has PD, although it often seems that we have it together. EB

My first visit to a neurologist specializing in movement disorders was on April 7, 2008.

I remember the moment well. It was my sixty-fourth birthday. The doctor greeted me with a handshake and ushered me into her office, which was plain and sparsely furnished. She asked me some questions, watched me walk briefly, tested my balance with a few unexpected tugs from behind, took one arm and then the other, and appeared to listen as she cranked them around at the elbows. I thought, *what on earth are you looking for?*

"Cogwheeling," she said as if hearing my thought.

Cogwheeling, of course! What is that?

She asked if my handwriting had been changing. I immediately pictured Leslie, the school secretary, squinting at the little yellow Post-it notes I passed along to her. They looked like blue ant tracks, walking erratically along the thin lines. Yes, my handwriting was shrinking.

"Have you been reading about Parkinson's disease?" the doctor asked. Before I could respond, she added, "You have a textbook case."

We talked a few minutes longer. I learned that I was at the typical age for the disease to appear; in fact, it had likely been with me, undiagnosed, for twenty years or more. The disease has no cure, but it is not fatal. (I wasn't sure that was good news or not.) I learned that there are various medications available to manage the disease, though nothing has been found to halt or reverse it. And "managing" the disease is not a simple matter. Please, doctor, tell us how to manage a small boat in a strong, unpredictable storm.

After the initial shock of hearing, "Yes, you have Parkinson's disease," I began to ask what I needed to do. There was no way to erase the diagnosis. The doctor was not going to call and say, "Sorry, we confused your file with another patient's. You really have Osgood -Slatter disease. It can be cured in two months." No, I had heard that diagnosis in seventh grade, when one knee was swollen and sore. Truth be told, until recently I had always been extraordinarily healthy. "Fit as a fiddle," my mother would say.

We hear many folks declare they are "fighting" cancer, in one form or another, and we respond with and sympathy and support. Yes, cancer is a scourge, to be resisted on every front. We treat it as an enemy, and I understand why. Ten years ago I had a dangerously high PSA level and decided to have my prostate removed. It was the right decision, as the surgery revealed. The doctor was concerned that the cancer might spread to my bladder. I was monitored carefully for several years and can say I escaped. There doesn't seem to be that option with PD. We can't approach it as an enemy but must seek ways to work with it, to search how it lives in us, even what it can teach us.

For most of us, PD exerts a relentless pressure toward contraction: a gradual, unforgiving sense of diminishment, as if one's subtle body were shrinking. Imagine a towel being wrung out, or a vise slowly closing within. It is not just the rigidity in our movement and posture; there are tremors for many, the unwelcome, erratic, jerky motions called dyskinesia as the side effect of long-term use of key medications and the ongoing struggle to find the most effective forms of medication and physical exercise. For some, and here I include myself, there is a corresponding loss or slowing of our ability to express our thoughts and feelings.

It is hard not to feel overwhelmed. So far, I can still find comfort in a kind hug or a good night's sleep, only to wake and realize my body is not the one I remember — once so flexible and obedient, so able to do my wishes. But the disease progresses; it really is, as they say, "chronic and degenerative." So how can I pretend there is hope here? Am I kidding myself? Let's be real.

Claire's response to this internal dialogue has been urgent and clear: "Remember, the disease is *not* you." Early on I heard the same advice coming from a wise and dear friend at work: "So, you have PD; but the PD is *not* you." That distinction has become central in my understanding of the challenge I face every day. At my core, I am whole and well.

In the second year after my diagnosis, I began to view PD as a condition, an entity, almost a being, that had come into my life and intended to stay. I saw it as an "uninvited guest" in our home. It

120

wouldn't be pushed out. It took up little space at first, yet its presence was undeniable. It adjusted to our routines, it hid in various medications, it was everywhere and nowhere. Sometimes it seemed to sleep—can we relax now? Other times it shook my arms, grabbed control of my legs, turned my walking into a stagger. My hands, those faithful assistants in the woodworking and carving I love to do, grew stiff and clumsy.

The non-motor symptoms of PD began to come forward, too: deep fatigue, spells of confusion, unexpected difficulties with speech, making conversation with Claire harder for both of us. In those moments, I would feel my mind searching for the word I wanted, as my tongue stumbled awkwardly around trying to form the right sound. *Was the Uninvited Guest playing games with us?* I confused dates, needed reminders about medication, and often felt pulled down by a general sense of loss or diminishment. Claire sometimes wondered where I was, what I was doing—and so did I.

I marveled how others with PD kept going. I saw an old friend with PD recently and asked, "How goes?" He indicated things were pretty steady for him. With the help of his neurologist (the same one I have) he was managing to do all he wanted to do. He had found a sweet spot in the balancing of medication, exercise, and attitude that was working. I was glad for him, but I must confess I longed for the same stability.

Now, after the first decade of our journey with PD, the disease is visible in my walk, my posture, my face, and those who know PD recognize it immediately. I find more people asking me very sincerely, "How are you doing?" My response, equally sincere, is, "The disease is progressing, and so am I."

And how have I been "progressing"? Early on, I discovered four areas in which to challenge the Uninvited Guest. They are not new or unique, but they describe our struggle for hope in the stormy seas ahead. We engage each with an eagerness to grow and learn, and share what we find along the way.

Medication
Physical activity
Care and companionship
Faith

Medication

Finding one's way through the maze of available medications for PD has proven more complicated than I had expected. One thing seems clear: Each person's path through that maze is different. What works for me may not work for you. We soon discovered that an experienced neurologist with training in movement disorders would be an essential player on our PD team, and we found one fairly close to home in rural western Massachusetts. Her approach to my condition was thoughtful and measured, which Claire and I appreciated. She observed my symptoms over several visits, and then gradually introduced small doses of Sinemet, a blend of carbidopa and levodopa, long regarded as the gold standard medication for PD. It made a real difference in the early years. Many days I felt close to normal, and I could walk for miles.

With time, Claire and I felt the need for a neurologist based in a larger practice, which we found at a major hospital, almost two hours away. Our new neurologist brought deeper experience with the disease and an immediate awareness of the latest options for treatment. We had wide-ranging conversations about the disease, and we recently embarked on a new, more powerful formulation of the early medication I had been on. It felt a bit like driving a new car. Such power! And such an intimidating list of possible side effects! It seems to be helping, and when I am exactly on time with my dosage three times each day, side effects like dyskinesia are less and I welcome the strength of the medication. But it does leave me wondering who is in charge here—me, or that familiar presence, the Uninvited Guest. Is there a simpler and more natural way to stay afloat?

Physical Activity

Exercise! That is the essential, natural complement to the prevailing emphasis on medication for every person with PD. As Claire has written, I have always loved to walk and hike, and I do that every day I can. I see walking as the archetypical exercise for all of us, with PD or not. Especially if one does it consciously, with attention to the whole body in motion, legs stretching forward, posture upright, arms swinging in a reciprocating rhythm, outside if possible, you just know it is good for you! But I must add a word of caution: Parkinson's can be downright ornery. After a decade of devoted walking to manage my symptoms, I have recently been seized by episodes of severe festination, during which

I lose control of my pace and stumble forward, faster and faster.

Fortunately there are many other ways to exercise. One ninety year old doctor told me soon after I was diagnosed, "You will get advice to exercise in this way or that by all kinds of experts, but the best exercise is the one you most like to do. Build your program around it! That will keep you going!" In my experience, a variety of exercises is most helpful, from Dance for PD to walking, rowing, cycling, and highly-structured routines like the Community Wellness Program for People with Parkinson's Disease, developed by a dedicated team at the Center for Neurorehabilitation at Boston University. (www.bu.edu.neurorehab) There are also specific exercises to strengthen one's voice, hands, balance, even sense of humor. As I see it, vigorous exercise of all sorts works to expand us, to enliven us, and thereby to counter the forces of contraction so persistent in PD. I recently joined a singing class for people with PD, and we sing our hearts out. The lively young teacher remarked, "Singing is an athletic activity too".

Care and Companionship

The Parkinson's path runs through all sorts of emotions, from spells of depression and despair to bursts of delight with the simplest gestures of kindness and support. While dramatic improvements in medical treatments will come and better understanding of alternative approaches will take hold, the need for caregivers will remain. The disease calls out for others to help: "I can't do this on my own!" Claire has recognized this need for help from the day of my diagnosis, if not before! (Come to think of it, she kissed me first; that was the beginning of her care, fifty-two years ago.) I'm sure many couples, as they reckon with the advance of PD, find that the one without PD becomes the caregiver, out of devotion or necessity or both. It is a hard role to sustain, and for those who no longer have a spouse or partner it must be unbearable. I regard the people who take on the role of caregiver as genuine heroes. Then there are volunteers who literally *give* their care to support others, with no expectation of personal gain. Beyond generosity, I feel PD can evoke a spirit of empathy in those who understand deeper challenges of the disease day after day. I am deeply moved by the kindness of heart so readily offered. When I look around in my little world, I find companionship from family, friends, co-workers, kindred spirits, and I am very grateful. But I also know that isolation and loneliness often accompany PD as it advances, and we may find ourselves being comforted with companionship from unexpected places. As I sit quietly in prayer, sometimes I hear the words come: "You are not alone."

Faith

If you haven't noticed, the Uninvited Guest can bring us to our knees. It has the knack of challenging us with fundamental questions, whether we are ready for them or not. Why did I get PD? Where do I find the courage to meet it, not just now but over the years ahead, when symptoms usually intensify? Is there some message in this for me? I've been told there is always cause for gratitude—even now? And what about my wonderful wife, and our family? Did they ask for this? The questions provoke all kinds of responses, from despair and denial to hope and confidence that all is well. But from my perspective, the questions can all be reduced to one: Where is my faith?

Let me answer by showing you a picture of a carving I created around the time of my PD diagnosis, ten years ago. Little did I know at that time what big waves *we* would be subject to. It is my attempt to illustrate a moment in the Gospels when Jesus was crossing a lake in a small boat with several of his disciples. Jesus lay down in the bow of the boat and fell asleep. His disciples were in the back when suddenly a fierce storm arose, huge waves threatened to crash into the boat and swamp it. Still, Jesus slept. The disciples were terrified, and woke Jesus, "Help us, we're drowning!" He stood, told the storm to be still, and the lake was instantly calm.

Jesus then asked his disciples, "Where is your faith?" They were in awe of his strength. I felt that awe when working on this sculpture. I see in the figure of Jesus the essential core of every person. That is a light, a part of the divine light pervading all creation. When we align with that spirit within us, we become calm, yet strong; we have found faith.

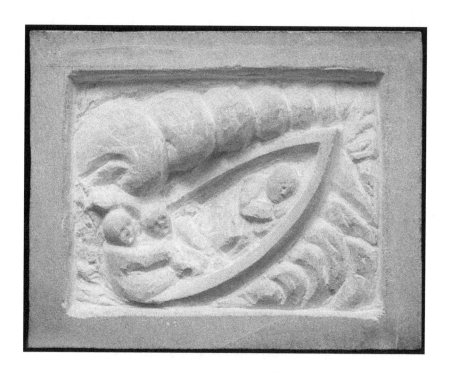

Claire and I pray for strength and understanding. So far, we are keeping afloat. In our quiet time together almost every morning, we face the realities of Parkinson's disease as faithfully as we can. We thank the spiritual world for all we have been given in the fifty years of our marriage, remind each other of the ways we are continually blessed, and call out the innate power of our individual sovereignty, the essential dignity and divinity of our beings. We are still whole, no matter the storms and trials that come with PD.

Ten Books in Our Boat

Many are the books that have helped us. The complete list is much too long, so we trimmed it down to the ten titles we've reached for most frequently these past ten years. Here they are:

Guides on our Parkinson's journey

The Brain's Way of Healing: Remarkable Discoveries and Recoveries from the Frontiers of Neuroplasticity, by Norman Doidge, M.D. (Viking Press, 2015)

Navigating Life with Parkinson's Disease, by Sotirios Parashos and Ruth Wichmann with Todd Melby (Oxford University Press, 2013)

Brain Storms: The Race to Unlock the Mysteries of Parkinson's Disease, by Jon Palfreman (Farrar, Straus & Giroux, 2015)

Parkinson's Disease: *A Complete Guide for Patients & Families*, by William J. Weiner, M.D., Lisa M. Shulman, M.D., and Anthony E. Lang, FRCP (2nd edition) (John Hopkins University Press, 2007)

Every Victory Counts: Essential Information and Inspiration for a Lifetime of Wellness with Parkinson's Disease, by Monique Giroux, M.D., and Sierra Farris, PA-C, MPAS (Davis Phinney Foundation for Parkinson's)

Guides on our spiritual journey

Meditations on Christ, by Lee Irwin (Lorian Press, 2016)

Open Mind, Open Heart, by Thomas Keating (Continuum Publishing Company, 1992)

How to Know Higher Worlds, by Rudolf Steiner (Anthroposophic Press, 1994)

Subtle Worlds: An Explorer's Field Notes, by David Spangler (Lorian Press, 2010)

Turning: Words Heard from Within (Anthroposophic Press, 1994)

And one wonderful film

"Capturing Grace," an extraordinary performance by the Mark Morris Dance Group and people with Parkinson's, featuring Dave Iverson, a journalist and filmmaker who himself has been diagnosed with PD (Passion River Productions)

Acknowledgements

Thank you to the skilled and generous professionals who have helped us in so many ways: Rani Athreya MD, Amanda Bernhard, Tami DeAngelis, Debra Ellis, Laurence Klein MD, Steven Lee MD, Lisa Moore, Diana O'Brien, Fritha Pengelly, Shelley Roberts.

Thank you to two wonderfully persistent and exacting word-loving friends who helped shaped this book: Ruth Carney and Thea Welch. Thanks also to our other cheer-readers: Karen Foss, Michael Lipson, Leslie Luchonok, Kathryn Mcavoy, Molly Scherm, Debbie Shriver.

Thank you to our PD pals: Maureen Flannery, Peggy Gurman, James Heflin, Ed O'Neil, Richard Parmett, Richard Pree, Claude Pepin, Steve McCarthy, John Mcavoy, Andrea Wright.

Thank you always and forever Laurel, Christa, Bernie, Thor and our grandchildren, Ellie, Freya, Lulu and Wynn.

Thank you Jeremy Berg for your warm and quick "Yes!" to our story.

And thank you David Spangler for being such an encouraging, inspiring and tender friend.